Ophthalmic Anesthesia

OPHTHALMIC ANESTHESIA

James P. Gills, MD
St. Lukes Cataract and Laser Institute
Tarpon Springs, Florida

Robert F. Hustead, MD
Ochsner Eye Center
Wichita, Kansas

Donald R. Sanders, MD, PhD
Center for Clinical Research
Chicago, Illinois

Medical Writer
Leslie Bendra Sabbagh

SLACK Incorporated, 6900 Grove Road, Thorofare, New Jersey 08086-9447

SLACK International Book Distributors

Japan
Igaku-Shoin, Ltd.
Tokyo International P.O. Box 5063
1-28-36 Hongo, Bunkyo-Ku
Tokyo 113
Japan

Canada
McGraw-Hill Ryerson Limited
300 Water Street
Whitby, Ontario
L1N 9B6

In all other regions throughout the world, SLACK professional reference books are available through offices and affiliates of McGraw-Hill, Inc. For the name and address of the office serving your area, please correspond to

McGraw-Hill, Inc.
Medical Publishing Group
Attn: International Marketing Director
1221 Avenue of the Americas —28th Floor
New York, NY 10020
(212)-512-3955 (phone)
(212)-512-4717 (fax)

Editorial Director: Cheryl D. Willoughby
Publisher: Harry C. Benson

Ophthalmic anesthesia / [edited by] James Gills, Robert Hustead, Donald Sanders.
  p. cm
  Includes bibliographical references and index.
  ISBN 1-55642-214-8 (Hard) :
  1. Anesthesia in ophthalmology. I. Gills, James P., II. Hustead, Robert, III. Sanders, Donald R.
  [DNLM: 1. Anesthesia,   2. Eye--surgery.]
RE82.063   1993
617.9′677--dc20
DCL
for Library of Congress   92-49304

Printed in the United States of America

Published by: SLACK Incorporated
                6900 Grove Road
                Thorofare, NJ 08086-9447

Last digit is print number: 10   9   8   7   6   5   4   3   2   1

Special Credit and Acknowledgment

Bergen, Michael P., *Vascular Architecture in the Human Orbit*, Swets and Zeitlinger, BV, Lisse, 1982. Figures: 1.10, 1.11, 1.26 (1.41c), 1.32, 1.33 (1.47c), 1.45c, 1.46c, 1.55.

Bloomberg "Anterior Periocular Anesthesia: Five Years Experience" *J Cataract Refract Surgery* 1991, Vol 17, 508-511. Figures 3.2 - 3.8.

Davis, David, "Peribulbar Anesthesia" *Ophthalmology Clinics of North America*, Vol 3, No. 1 March 1990, Pages 105-107. Figures: 3.9-3.12.

de Jong, RH, *Local Anesthetics*, Second Edition, Charles C. Thomas, Springfield, 1977, p 51-62. Figures: 2.1-2.9.

Dixon, Cheryl, "The Sprotte, Whitacre and Quincke Spinal Needles," *Anesthesia Review*, Vol 18, Sept/Oct 1991. Becton-Dickinson, Rutherford, NJ. Figure: 3.1.

Gills, James, "A Technique of Retrobulbar Block with Paralysis of Orbitus Oculi", *J Cataract Surgery*, 1983, Vol 9, pages 339-340. Figures: 3.12, 3.14.

Koornneef, Leo, "Eyelid and Orbital Fascial Attachments and their Clinical Significance", *Eye*, Volume 2, Professional and Scientific Publishers, London, 1988. Figure: 1.15.

Koornneef, Leo, "Orbital Bony and Soft Tissue Anatomy" from *The Eye and the Orbit in Thyroid Disease*, editors CA Gorman et al, Raven Press, New York, 1984. Figures: 1.12, 1.36 (1.48c), 1.37 (1.51c), 1.39, 1.52 (1.40).

Koornneef, Leo, *Spatial Aspects of Orbital Musculo-Fibrous Tissue in man*, Swets and Zeitlinger, BV, Amsterdam and Lisse, 1977. Figures: 1.4, 1.5, 1.6, 1.14, 1.27 (1.41d), 1.28 (1.42d), 1.30 (1.44c), 1.31 (1.45d), 1.35 (1.47d), 1.42c, 1.43c, 1.43d, 1.44d, 1.46d, 1.53, 1.58.

Koornneef, Leo, Schmidt ED, Van Der Gaag, R. "The Orbit: Structure, Autoantigens and Pathology." Wall JR, How, J, editors, *Graves' Ophthalmology: Current Issues in Endocrinology and Metabolism*. Blackwell Scientific Publications, Boston, 1990. Figures: 1.29, 1.34, 1.56.

Kozoil J, "Anatomy of the Orbit" Peyman, Sanders and Goldberg, editors *Principles and Practice of Ophthalmology*. WB Saunders, Philadelphia, 1980. Figure: 1.57.

Paulter, SE, Grizzard, WS, et al. "Blindness from Retrobulbar Injection into the Optic Nerve," *Ophth Surg*, 1989, Vol 17, p 334-337. Figures: 118, 119.

Reinecke, Robert, editor, chapter "Ophthalmic Anesthesia" by WS Grizzard, *Ophthalmology Annual*, Raven Press, New York, 1989. Figures: 1.9 (3.16, 4.1), 3.20.

Vogl, G., "Stereotactic Retrobulbar Anesthesia Using CT" *J Computer Assisted Tomography*, Vol 14, Raven Press, New York, 1990. Figures: 1.60, 1.61.

Wang, "Peribulbar Anesthesia for Ophthalmic Procedures" , *J Cataract Surgery*, 1988, Vol 14, p 441-443. Figure: 3.18.

Zonneveld, FW, *Computed Tomography of the Temporal Bone and Orbit*, Urban & Swartzenberg, Munich, Germany, 1987. Figures: 41a,b-52a,b.

CONTENTS

One ANATOMY

Robert F. Hustead, MD; Leo Koorneef, MD, PhD;
Frans W. Zonneveld, MD, PhD

Two PHARMACOLOGY

Robert F. Hustead, MD; Robert C. Hamilton MB, BCh

CONTRIBUTING AUTHORS

Leroy B. Bloomberg, MD
Bloomberg Eye Center
Newark, Ohio

David B. Davis II, MD
Medical Surgical Center
Hayward, California

Richard A. Fichman, MD
Fichman Eye Center
Manchester, Connecticut

Anibal Galindo, MD, PhD
Cedars Medical Center
Coral Gables, Florida

James P. Gills, MD
St. Luke's Cataract and Laser Insitute
Tarpon Springs, Florida

W. Sanderson Grizzard, MD
Family Medical Arts Center
Tampa, Florida

Robert C. Hamilton, MB, BCh
Gimbel Eye Centre
Calgary, Alberta, Canada

Robert F. Hustead, MD
Ochsner Eye Center
Wichita, Kansas

Robert M. Kershner, MD
Orange Grove Eye Surgery Center
Tucson, Arizona

Leo Koornneef, MD, PhD
Orbita Centrum
Amsterdam, The Netherlands

Thomas Loyd, PA
St. Luke's Cataract and Laser Institute
Tarpon Springs, Florida

Mark R. Mandel, MD
Medical Surgical Eye Center
Hayward, California

Jaswant Singh Pannu, MD
Pannu Eye Institute
Fort Lauderdale, Florida

Jeffrey G. Straus, MD
Straus/Azar Medical Surgical
     Laser Eye Center
Metairle and Gretna, Louisiana

Spencer P. Thornton, MD
Baptist Hospital
Nashville, Tennessee

Hai-Shiuh Wang, MD
Eye Care Associates
Youngstown, Ohio

Charles H. Williamson, MD
Williamson Eye Center
Baton Rouge, Louisiana

Frans W. Zonneveld, MD, PhD
University Hospital Utrecht
Utrecht, The Netherlands

PREFACE

This book is the result of a concerted effort to provide new anatomic and pharmacologic insights to the clinician, anesthetist, and researcher on the state of ophthalmic anesthesia today.

The MRI, CT and cryosection images show for the first time the definitive anatomy of the globe and orbit; the relationship of orbital and skeletal structures; and individual variability. This new knowledge provided the impetus for the book. But ultimately, it was the collaboration of an international group of anatomists, ophthalmologists, anesthesiologists, and clinicians who gave unstintingly of their experience and knowledge that brought this book to print. The relatively recent development of topical anesthesia as an effective alternative to ocular anesthetic injections is also included in an effort to provide ophthalmologists with the most timely information currently available.

We hope that all clinicians will draw from the shared knowledge and new insights discussed here to provide more efficacious and safe ophthalmic anesthesia for their patients.

ACKNOWLEDGMENTS

The editors wish to express gratitiude to the Orbita Centrum University of Amsterdam, the Netherlands for making available anatomical preparations and illustrations used in the Anatomy chapter and Duane Penner of Slide Graphics, Wichita, Kansas for preparation of the computer graphics used in the illustrations.

The editors would like to thank Dr. Hustead's wife, Joy, and two daughters, Barbara and Judy, for their work in preparation of the manuscript.

The editors are grateful to the St. Luke's Cataract and Laser Institute, Tarpon Springs, Florida, for financial grants toward the cost of illustrations and preparation.

One

Robert F. Hustead, MD
Leo Koornneef, MD, PhD
Frans W. Zonneveld, MD, PhD

ANATOMY

Introduction*

This chapter describes topographical anatomy, anatomy of the bony orbit, the geometric relationships of the globe and orbit, and the spatial relationships of the globe to orbital structures. Also discussed are the septal compartments through which needles must pass, extraocular muscles, the relationship of arteries, veins, and nerves, orbital adipose tissue compartments, and the unique character of the orbit and its nerves that make orbital regional anesthesia so different from regional anesthesia in other parts of the body. Familiarity with anatomy is essential to those doing their first orbital injection of local anesthetic—or to those who wish to improve this skill.

Orbital anatomy for regional anesthesia is usually learned from artists' drawings, (Figure 1.1) or observation of a skull. For those who wish to thoroughly pursue the topic, procurement of an atlas and a skull is advised in addition to perusing the photographs of the skull shownin Figure 1.2. Computer graphics have been generated from photographs of this skull to facilitate spatial visualization of the orbital structures and their associated nerves, arteries, and veins (Figure 1.3).

Unfortunately, as descriptive as the graphics and artists' drawings are in learning names, this method is of limited value for those learning to inject local anesthetic into the orbit to block sensory and motor nerves.

Those desiring to improve their current technique or to explain "clinically unsatisfactory blocks" benefit from reviewing diagrams and drawings, as above, but they must be familiar with the spatial relationships of the structures to be blocked and with the connective tissue of the orbit which directs the flow of anesthetic after it leaves the needle.

This chapter presents spatial orbital anatomy the same way the needle travels during blocks and combines photographs of live persons with cadaver specimens to establish the spatial relationships of structures to supporting connective tissue. All references and photographs are of the right orbit and globe, except when noted.

Throughout this chapter, the editors have used abbreviations on the figures to indicate certain anatomic structures. Please refer to the Guide to Figure Abbreviations located on page 205 for definitions.

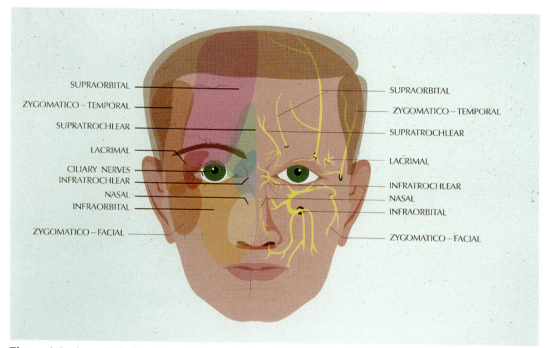

Figure 1.1. An artist's drawing of the sensory areas of the eye and orbit on the right and the sensory nerves on the left. The sensory areas of the conjunctiva and lids show great overlap clinically. It is necessary to block both nerves of an overlap area to produce sensory anesthesia.

The histologic specimens and spatial reconstructions reviewed in this chapter were prepared by Leo Koornneef, MD, PhD[1-6] and have been combined with cryosection technique to validate structures seen with computed tomography of the orbit by Frans Zonneveld, MD, PhD.[7-9]

Analysis of such specimens promotes visualization of the exact structures through which the needle passes; the nerves into which anesthetic must diffuse; and the connective tissue that forms the fascial planes along which anesthetic will spread. These planes are a factor in anesthetic effectiveness because they limit diffusion.[10]

Leo Koornneef has taught orbital anatomy both as an anatomist and ophthalmologist.[11] He is currently in the active practice of oculoplastic, lacrimal, and orbital surgery. As a surgeon with orbital and septal familiarity, he now manipulates the septa and the adipose compartments, and is able to see how the tissue vary in different persons.

Background

Koornneef attempted to resolve four clinical problems involving anatomy by the surgical dissection of fresh cadaver orbits:

• Why do blow out fractures of the inferior orbital floor cause diplopia due to limited upward movement of the eye during upward gaze?

• Why does dissection in the orbit to repair orbital floor fractures often cause acute venous congestion in the orbit?

• Why does injection of radio-opaque material into the "retrobulbar space" occasionally lead to blindness?

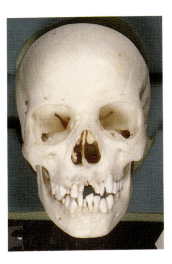

Figure 1.2a. Frontal view. In a forward view, the openings of both optic foramina along the nasal edge of the orbit are barely visible. The optic foramen cannot be entered from the infero-nasal quadrant, whereas the supero-nasal makes an unobstructed path. Note the superior and inferior orbital fissures and the spine where the lateral rectus muscle attaches at the lateral edge of the superior orbital fissure.

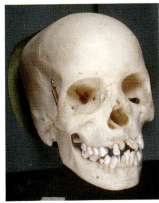

Figure 1.2b. Frontal view of the right orbit along the orbital axis. The optic foramen and the supraorbital fissure are quite visible. The orbital apex gives a different perspective, as the optic canal is anterior and nasal to the actual apex which is the strut of the sphenoid bone. The concept of the orbital apex must be visualized by those doing nerve blocks because it is referred to in so many descriptions of anatomy and anesthesia technique.

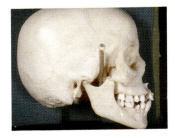

Figure 1.2c. Profile or sagittal view. The superior orbital rim is posterior to the inferior orbital rim; note how laterally the inferior orbital rim sweeps posteriorly. Note the opening of the naso-lacrimal canal. Most CT scans and histologic sections use the sagittal plane of the orbital axis.

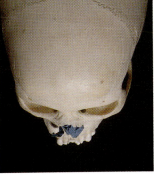

Figure 1.2d. Top, horizontal, or transverse view. The lacrimal canal is anterior to the superior orbital rim. The most anterior topographical feature is the inferior orbital rim at the zygomatic/maxillary suture. This is 3 mm medial to the junction of the medial 2/3 and lateral 1/3 of the inferior rim.

Figure 1.2. The skull of a young caucasian of medium orbital and facial structure, probably female. The skull has a "retrobulbar path length" of 47 mm which corresponds to the median of the Katsev data, described in Figure 1.17. The skull has two anomalies, a deviated nasal septum and an anomalous supraorbital foramen. Instead of a common supraorbital foramen or notch, there is a foramen for each of the medial and lateral branches which divided in the orbit and exited through corresponding foramina. The supraorbital artery exited through the lateral foramen. Review Figure 1.25 for nomenclature of anatomic planes. There are iatragenic fractures of the ethmoid bone.

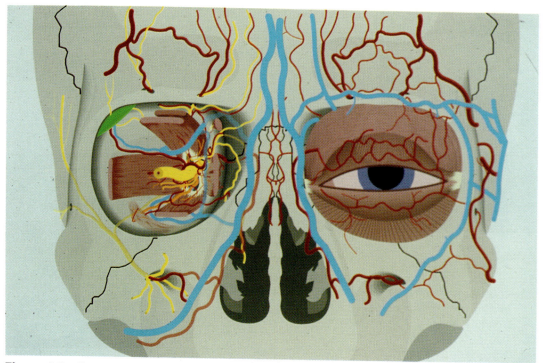

Figure 1.3. Computer-generated graphics of the skull in Figure 1.2. In the right orbit the extraocular muscles, the optic nerve, veins, arteries, and nerves are in true coronal perspective in primary gaze. Point of focus is 5 mm behind the hind surface of the eye. Nerves are yellow, the muscles brownish-red, the arteries bright red, and the veins bright blue; structures in canals are silhouetted. The veins and arteries anterior to the hind surface of the globe are lighter shades.

Note the long path of the inferior branch of the ophthalmic artery that goes to the inferior oblique muscle and the associated branch of the oculomotor nerve. The long course takes the structure along the floor of the orbit along the lateral surface of the inferior rectus muscle. In 80% of persons, the ophthalmic artery crosses superior to the optic nerve, as in the figure; in the other 20%, however, the ophthalmic artery crosses underneath the optic nerve where it is much more vulnerable to injury with needles directed toward the orbital apex from the floor of the orbit.

The left orbit and lids with superficial arteries and veins of the face and lids are depicted. The reader should visualize the more vascular areas of the lids and orbit to minimize risk of hemorrhage or hematoma. The least vascular pathways into the orbit follow (ATCs) adispose tissue components.

All structures will be named as they appear later in histologic sections or reconstructions; the arteries and veins are named in Figure 1.10.

• How do sub-Tenon's injections of local anesthetic present as fullness of the upper eyelids?

An unexpected discovery was made when the orbit was dissected through the conjunctiva into the fascia anterior to the equator of the globe—there existed extensive radial connective tissue or septa (Figures 1.4, 1.5, and 1.6). These radial septa continued posterior to the equator, therefore, histologic thin sections, special thick sections, and three-dimensional orbital reconstruction were necessary to demonstrate the septa because careful surgical dissection proved too destructive.

Radial connective tissue septa support the globe and attach it to the extraocular

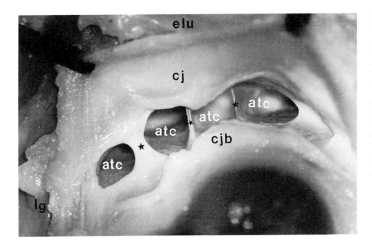

Figure 1.4. Incision of the conjunctiva of the superior fornix reveals connective tissue strands between frontal periorbit and Tenon's capsule. Stars or asterisks indicate connective tissue strands or septa throughout this chapter. Adipose tissue compartments (ATCs) are labelled; they occur between septal walls. (With permission from Swets & Zeitlinger BV)

Figure 1.5. Connective tissue septa between the lacrimal bone periorbit and Tenon's capsule. Stars or asterisks indicate connective tissue septa. ATCs are labelled. (With permission from Swets & Zeitlinger BV)

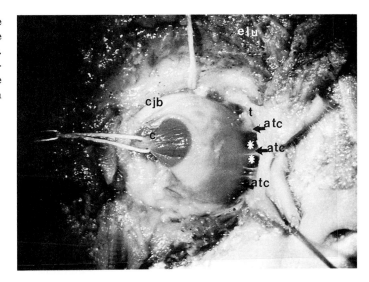

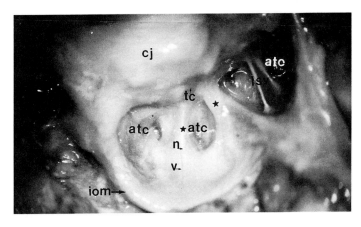

Figure 1.6. Septa between Tenon's capsule and the inferior oblique muscle. Some septa carry vessels or nerves, or both. Stars or asterisks indicate septa. ATCs are labelled. (With permission from Swets & Zeitlinger BV)

muscles and to the periorbit. This connective tissue divides the orbit into four major anterior to posterior connective tissue compartments, which will be discussed later in the chapter and appear as Figure 1.53;[5,12] one compartment is associated with each of the rectus muscles. A closed surgical inner space or "retrobulbar space" could not be distinguished.[12,13] Adipose tissue compartments containing many septa are associated with each of the muscle connective tissue compartments. This organization of the orbital connective tissue develops in the third fetal month.[3,6]

The septal compartments vary in size and compliance in different persons [14-17] and have been confirmed in living persons at surgery.[18,19] The septa, which form the walls of the compartments, contain collagen fibers, elastic fibers, and some contain smooth muscle.[4] The septa vary as to tensile strength and elasticity—or compliance. Throughout the chapter the term compliance will be used because it denotes mathematically and semantically that the septa can be stretched with varying amounts of pressure or tension. The more compliant, the more easily they are stretched.

The connective tissue septa attach the globe and extraocular muscles to the periorbit, coordinate motion of the muscles and the optic nerve, provide support for the venous system of the orbit as shown in Figure 1.11b, and provide cogent anatomic explanation to the above questions:

The complex of the inferior rectus/inferior oblique is attached to itself, to the globe, and to the periorbit by septa—all of which gets trapped in blowout fractures.[6,19]

The veins of the orbit are easily compressed during orbital dissection because they are suspended in the walls of the septal compartments.[6]

The compliance of the septa and septal compartments varies with different individuals; pressure adequate to compress the arteries and veins can be achieved during orbitography by rapid injection into small or non-compliant compartments.[6]

The continuity of the septal compartments of Tenon's capsule with the connective tissue of the lids produces a pathway for fluids to dissect from behind the eye into the lids; thus, anesthetic injected in the sub-Tenon's space or the retrobulbar space can end up in the lids in some individuals. Anesthetic injected posterior to the orbital septum can follow these same pathways to block the lids.[6]

Additional analysis of specimens further explains problems encountered in orbital regional anesthesia:

- Can safer pathways for needles be easily determined by visualizing the structures through which needles pass?
- What reference points will provide optimal safety for needle insertion and effectiveness of anesthetic injection?
- What is the "retrobulbar space" and what is the muscle cone? Why does the muscle cone retain anesthetic injection? What are the escape routes?
- How much space exists between the muscles to allow anesthetic to exit the muscle cone for the periorbital areas, and by what routes does injection in the periorbit enter the retrobulbar space?
- What factors determine whether anesthetic flows anteriorly to block the lids or follows the epidural space to the chiasm?
- Why do needles placed in similar loci in the orbit followed by injection of similar volume of anesthetic produce total anesthesia and akinesia in one patient and almost no block in another? Does this failure to produce akinesia arise from the failure to penetrate the septa between the inferior rectus and the lateral rectus (as is usually taught) or is it failure of anesthetic to enter an "oculomotor compartment?"

- Why should bulbar chemosis be a regular feature of "periocular" blocks?
- Where are the best sites for injection of local anesthetic to produce lid akinesia or to produce anesthesia of the lids, without producing lid akinesia?

Analysis of the histologic sections and reconstructions of the orbit will allow the reader to visualize needle pathway from penetration of the skin to injection sites in the orbit and then to follow the spread of anesthetic in the orbit.

Understanding the trajectories and pathways of needles traversing the orbit is critically important to safety; understanding how the injectate behaves in the orbit is instrumental in achieving effective anesthesia.

Such knowledge will allow clinicians to avoid iatrogenic trauma, to better anticipate where anesthetic will go, to evaluate the anatomy of blocks, and to make supplemental injections in more anatomically desirable parts of the orbit to achieve safer, more effective blocks.

This chapter was written to familiarize the reader with the basic structure of the orbit, the real anatomical distances, and the variations seen in different individuals. Photographs, line drawings, and histologic sections in actual size are featured.

Topography and Variations

There are many variations in eyelid size, the size of the palpebral fissure, and the amount of fatty tissue in the lids anterior or posterior to the orbital septum. These factors influence the sites of injection, the safe passageways for needles, and effectiveness of anesthetic injected for lid blocks.

When the patient has very lax lids and a wide palpebral fissure (Figure 1.7) it is easy to use either a subconjunctival or percutaneous approach to the lids or orbit; lid blocks in such patients will require considerable volume of anesthetic.

When the patient has very tense lids and a narrow palpebral fissure (Figure 1.8) a subconjunctival approach can be difficult, except at the medial canthal angle. The preseptal space of tight lids accepts only a small volume of anesthetic and, therefore, can be blocked with a minimal volume of anesthetic, but the block may wear off quickly because of the small amount of anesthetic in the tissue.

Variations in lid structure and tension influence the route of the needle and are potentially important in the risk of globe penetration. The globe in Figure 1.8a could be perforated easily if the patient blinked or moved even slightly when the needle was in the lid or traversing the lid as it approached the equator of the eye. The orbicularis should be blocked first by preseptal injection of anesthetic, a separate nerve block, a block through the medial canthus (where squinting does not cause the needle to deviate), or a short general anesthetic to obviate squinting—this latter can engender problems of its own.

Forward set eyes and deep set eyes are common. The first patient, shown in Figure 1.7b, could be blocked from the inferotemporal approach readily because the equator of the eye is anterior to the inferior orbital rim. The equator of the deep set eye shown in Figure 1.8b is 7 mm behind the inferior orbital rim and there is considerable risk to the globe if the globe is large or the orbit is small. Fluid should be injected ahead of the needle in the capsulopalpebral fascia to create a safe passage past the equator in such patients. The lid should be open and the globe exposed so that contact of the needle with the sclera would give a visual as well as tactile signal to the anesthetist.

In Figure 1.7b the globe is concealed behind the superior orbital rim. This type of anatomy creates a hazardous route for a straight needle in the superior temporal

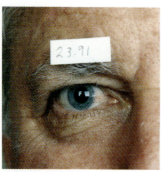

Figure 1.7a.

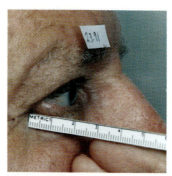

Figure 1.7b.

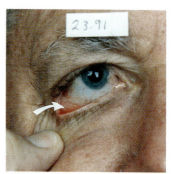

Figure 1.7c.

Figure 1.7. Patient with high brow, lax lids, wide palpebral fissure, and forward set globe. (a) Frontal view; (b) Sagittal view; (c) Frontal view with lid retracted laterally—note lax lids and herniation of the fat in Eisler's pocket (arrow). A needle inserted just posterior to the edge of the tarsal plate through this pocket will enter an ATC, anterior and lateral to the posterior lamella of the capsulopalpebral fascia (curved arrow), so that injection of local anesthetic in the mid-orbit will rarely cause chemosis. There is often a herniation of the orbital septum in this location, so that the needle will pass from the lid to the mid-orbit without touching any connective tissue structures .

Transconjunctival injection inferior to the tarsal plate into the preseptal space of the lid, anterior to the orbital septum, will block the sensory fibers to the lid and orbicularis. After penetrating the conjunctiva, the needle is directed toward the cheek with gentle flow of anesthetic; if the orbital septum is intact it will be felt as a "pop." Hydraulic dissection just anterior to the orbital septum in the pre-septal space will ensue.

quadrant. In Figure 1.8b the globe is well free of the superior orbital rim; if the orbit is generous, the supero-temporal approach may be optimum. Oriental patients often have deep set eyes, small orbits, small lids, and narrow palpebral fissures, but there is space in the extreme infero-lateral area to glide a needle with hydraulic dissection alongside the eye, although getting "behind the eye" may be dangerous. The medial compartment is always accessible in these patients.

Color Figures 1.7 and 1.8 provide a 3-D realization from the frontal plane as well as sagittally and allow good visualization of the structures and their relationships. Contrast this with Figure 1.9, a black and white rendition of the same area in an average eye. Such line drawings make it appear deceptively easy to slip a needle behind the globe when in many patients the task is difficult.

Examining and touching the facial structures, asking the patient to move the eye before a block, establishing any abnormalities of gaze and lack of tensile strength of the lids is extremely important.

The determination of individual variation is critical. It is the great variation in orbital structure and globe relationships that makes blocking the eye an art as well as a science.

Division of the Orbit Into Three Areas

Anesthesia technique is more readily visualized if the orbit is divided into three anterior-to-posterior spaces for better appreciation of the relationship of injection site, needle path, and the spaces into which the solution will flow, that is the anterior, the mid-, and the posterior orbit.

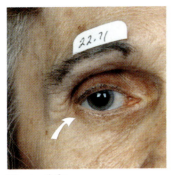

Figure 1.8a.

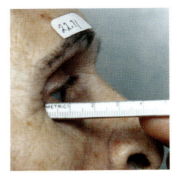

Figure 1.8b.

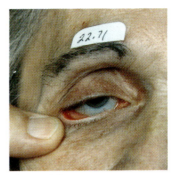

Figure 1.8c.

Figure 1.8. Patient with short, tight lids, and deep set globe. (a) Frontal view—arrow at site of transcutaneous puncture used by the author in "tight" lids. (b) Sagittal view—note how deep set the globe is. Perforation of the globe is easy in such deep set eyes using classical percutaneous or transconjunctival technique. A straight path adjacent to the periorbit just inferior to the lateral rectus muscle is available into the mid-orbit. Needle angulation toward the orbital apex could cause flexion of the needle, deviation of needle path, and potential perforation of the globe. (c) Note retraction of the lid does not cause eversion or exposure of Eisler's pocket, or the fornix of the conjunctival reflection. Such short lids are uncommon in caucasians, but common in orientals. A transcutaneous approach to the inferotemporal compartment (arrow) is easier than transconjunctival.

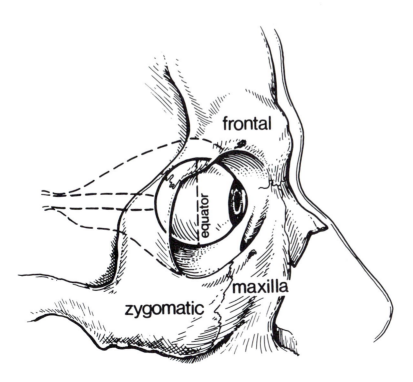

Figure 1.9. The equator of the eye is generally at, or slightly anterior to the lateral orbital rim. The position of the eye is variable, as seen in Figure 1.7 and 1.8, and must be assessed in each patient prior to injection. The eye is generally closer to the roof of the orbit than to the floor, and the frontal bone overhangs the eye making the inferotemporal approach the most open access to the retrobulbar space. (Reproduced with permission from WS Grizzard and Raven Press.)

This division is artificial because the globe, the extraocular muscles, and the septal compartments function as a unit[12] and there is no discrete division. However, this division should give no misinformation as does the erroneous concept that the space between the orbital septum and the optic canal can be divided into a "periorbital" space and a "retrobulbar" space.

The anterior orbit is primarily dense connective tissue with elastic fibers, smooth muscle, and minor adipose compartments. The mid-orbit is primarily muscle bellies, adipo-connective tissue, and the optic nerve. The posterior orbit consists primarily of origins of muscle, dense connective tissue, and a collection of arteries, nerves, and veins.

The anterior orbit, which is covered by the lids and conjunctiva, is the space between the lids and the sites of attachment of the extraocular muscles to the periorbit and sclera (2 to 5 mm anterior to the equator of the globe). This attachment region is a diffuse area of the "capsulopalpebral fascia" and ligaments. The anterior orbit is like a sponge with robust septal walls and adipose-filled chambers. The septa are primarily radial.

The intact orbital septum divides the anterior orbit into a pre- and a post-septal space. When the orbital septum is absent due to aging, trauma, or needle tracks, then communication between the orbit and the lids exists.

The mid-orbit begins anteriorly where the extraocular muscles and their septal continuations are attached to the periorbit or globe in the shape of a clover leaf indented by the muscles and ends posteriorly when the bellies of the extraocular muscles are very large in comparison to the adipose tissue between them, about 10 to 12 mm behind the hind surface of the globe.

The posterior orbit begins when the space between the extraocular muscles is less than one-half the breadth of the muscle, or at about 10 to 12 mm behind the hind surface of the globe; it ends at the optic canal. The space contained between the extraocular muscles in the posterior orbit is referred to as the "muscle cone."

The arteries run from the posterior orbit anteriorly where they anastomose with the extraorbital system (Figure 1.10a,b). The veins of the anterior orbit follow septa posteriorly (Figures 1.10c,d and 1.11a,b) to drain into the cavernous sinus.

Anatomy of the Anterior Orbit

The anterior orbit is characterized by many connective tissue septa attaching the globe and insertions of the extraocular muscles to the periorbit and to the lids shown in Figures 1.4, 1.5, & 1.6.[1,12] The septa in the anterior orbit are robust enough to resist dissection by a probe or dull needle, but stretchable so that they can be pulled out to double their length. Between the septa are small fat-filled compartments through which needles pass readily. Septa are anterior as well as posterior to the orbital septum and fat lobules pass through fenestrations in the orbital septum in the elderly. Anesthetics injected anterior or posterior to the orbital septum move through septal fenestrations to travel from one compartment to another. There are many fenestrations in the orbital septum in most specimens, and anesthetic, when injected posterior to it in great enough volume, can travel anteriorly through the fenestrations as well as along the needle track, thereby anesthetizing the skin and the overlying orbicularis muscle by blocking the nerve supply in the preseptal space.

Anesthetic in the preseptal space in adequate volume readily spreads to involve the entire lid and will often spread to both lids from a single injection site. The injection

Figure 1.10a. Spatial drawing of the arterial system in the human orbit seen in orbital axis perspective. This system emerges centrally from the top of the orbital cone, spreading radially to the periphery. Note the relatively fewer arteries in the area of the infero-nasal, infero-temporal, and supero-temporal ATCs. In this reconstructed series, the inferior muscular artery takes a lateral course in relation to the optic nerve instead of the more usual medial course. (Diameters of the vessels do not correspond exactly with reality.) (With permission from MP Bergen, MD and Swets & Zeitlinger BV)

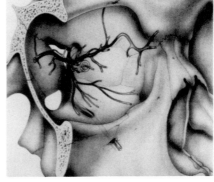

Fig 1.10a.

Figure 1.10b. Line diagram and names of the orbital arterial system. (With permission from MP Bergen, MD and Swets & Zeitlinger BV)

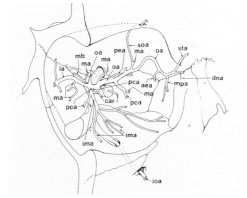

Fig. 1.10b.

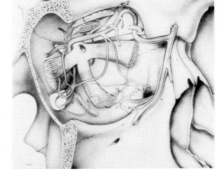

Fig. 1.10c

Figure 1.10c. Spatial drawing of the venous system in the human orbit. The veins form a complex of anastomosing vessels, creating a system of venous rings. In this reconstructed series no anterior collateral vein could be identified, whereas a double medial collateral vein is present.

Small veins in the infero-nasal compartment communicate with the facial vein anteriorly and the superior orbital vein posteriorly. Note the size of the superior ophthalmic vein in the supero-temporal quadrant, its tortuous course, and its many communications. It moves from 5 mm anterior of the hind surface of the eye in the supero-nasal quadrant, crossing obliquely at the hind surface of the eye and enters the supero-nasal compartment at or about 5-7 mm behind the hind surface. (With permission from MP Bergen, MD and Swets & Zeitlinger BV)

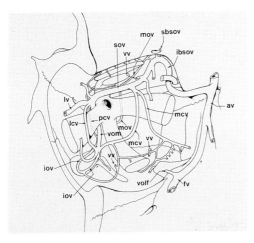

Figure 1.10d. Line diagram and names of the orbital venous system. (With permission from MP Bergen, MD and Swets & Zeitlinger BV—modified)

Figure 1.11a. Spatial drawing of the inter-relationships of the arterial and venous system with the septal complex of the inferior extrinsic eye muscles. The arteries radiating towards their target organs perforate the septa; the veins running circularly are confined to septa. (With permission from MP Bergen, MD and Swets & Zeitlinger BV—modified)

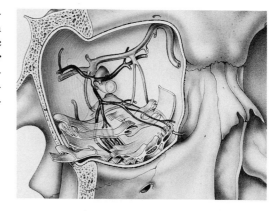

Figure 1.11b. Spatial drawing showing the inter-relationships of the two medial collateral veins, the superior ophthalmic vein (sov) and a muscular vein with the septal complex of the medial rectus muscle. on = optic nerve; * = connective tissue septa. (With permission from MP Bergen, MD and Swets & Zeitlinger BV)

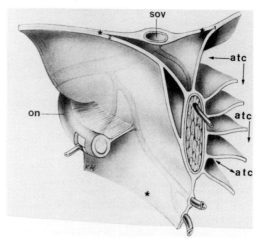

Figure 1.11c. A cleared section through an ATC from an area just above the orbital floor showing the micro-vessels arranged in loops. The septal walls contain only venules. The ATCs are rich in capillaries. The long micro-vessels tend to run in the long axis of ATCs. (With permission from MP Bergen, MD and Swets & Zeitlinger BV)

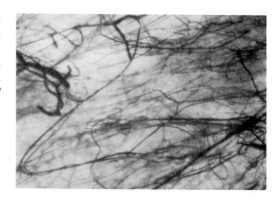

causes great pain if done rapidly; slow injection or painless solutions should be utilized.[62a,b]

The larger septa can be felt with the point of a sharp or dull needle and markedly resist penetration by dull needles (shown in Figures 1.4-1.6). If a septum is contacted, it is less traumatic to retract the needle and move it 0.5 to 1 mm rather than to bore through. When septa are avoided, one can move needles in the orbit with no motion of the globe or sensation on the part of the patient. Boring through cannot be distinguished from the needle penetrating a muscle, the globe, an artery, or vein—except by the disaster induced by damage. Since veins run in septal walls (Figure 11b), there is increased risk of bleeding if the septa are traumatized.

Septa vary in tensile strength; major septa form the walls of adipose tissue compartments (ATCs) (see also Figures 1.53a-d). Interiors of the ATCs are relatively avascular, "safe" pathways for needles, which can slide down the middle capillary beds of adipose compartments relatively easily (Figure 1.11c). The ciliary nerves and arteries are in the central ATC, close to the optic nerve where damage could occur from needle trauma.

The trochlear pulley and the reflected tendon of the superior oblique muscle are in the anterior orbit in the supero-nasal area (Figure 1.12) (see also Figure 1.36). Because of the delicate nature of the trochlea and the nearby blood vessels, this area is better avoided.

Safe Entrances to the Anterior Orbit

Needles entering the anterior orbit must be placed in avascular, atraumatic loci to avoid blood vessels in the lids and conjunctiva (shown in Figures 1.3 and 1.10), the canaliculi, and the trochlea. Deeper directed needles must miss septa, muscles, blood vessels, and nerves.

The adipose tissue compartments (ATCs) are natural entrance sites and tracts for entrance to the orbit. The ATCs will be marked with "ATC" or arrows on photographs of patients (Figures 1.13 and 1.14). In the right eye the ATCs are at 12:30-1:30, 2:30, 4:30, 7:30 to 8:00, and 10:45 and show bilateral symmetry. The ATCs are evident in the frontal section of the anterior orbit in Figure 1.14 and in all subsequent coronal histologic sections. The 12:30 site overlies the supraorbital artery and the superior ophthalmic vein and leads to a very vascular mid-orbital area, and is best avoided deeper than the anterior orbit. Even in the anterior area there are many veins, arteries, and nerves.

The percutaneous sites over the ATC at 2:30 and 4:30 may cause lid hematoma because of perforation of the palpebral arteries. The 4:30 site may injure the medial collateral vein (as shown in Figure 1.44d).

The 3:00-4:00 site, medial to the caruncle just posterior and lateral to the medial canthal fold, posterior to the medial canthal ligaments, is avascular and leads to a medial periconal ATC which communicates deeper with the 2:30 and 4:30 sites (as seen in Figures 1.25 and 1.26). The medial canthal fold (see small black arrow in Figure 1.12) is at 4:00 in most people, however, it can be from 2:30 to 4:30, and this must be considered in avoiding the medial rectus muscle which goes from 2:30 to 3:30.

A lateral entry area at 7:30-8:00 percutaneously or transconjunctivally has advantages over the much used 7:30-8:00 junction of the lateral 1/3 and medial 2/3 of the inferior orbital rim. This site has more space lateral to the globe, is more out of the patient's vision, and carries less risk of damage to the inferior oblique muscle or the oculomotor nerve and arterial branches to it (as shown in Figures 1.26 & 1.27); the nerve is visible lateral to the lateral rectus muscle. Furthermore, the lateral rectus muscle insertion on the globe can be seen as a reference, and a route inferior to it can be taken (small arrow—Figure 1.13a).

Figures 1.7c and 1.13b show the adipose compartment herniated below the tarsal plate where it can be entered transconjunctivally. This avascular adipose tissue compartment forms a tunnel alongside the equator parallel to the orbital axis, and is

Figure 1.12a. Schematic drawing of the extraocular muscles and globe. Cranial axial view after the orbital roof has been removed. Note the space between the muscle and the location of the trochlea. (With permission from Raven Press.)

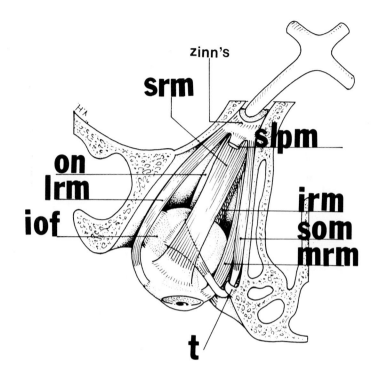

Figure 1.12b. Frontal view of globe and extraocular muscles to show relationship of trochlea and tendons of the superior oblique muscle, the space between the muscles, and the position and course of the inferior oblique muscle. (With permission from Raven Press.)

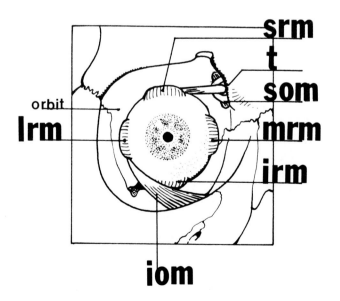

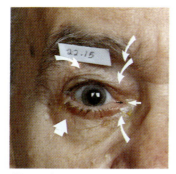

Figure 1.13a. Frontal view of patient with ATCs designated by arrows. Note the medial canthal angle at 4:00 (fine arrow) which makes an avascular immobile conduit for a needle to be placed in the medial ATC.

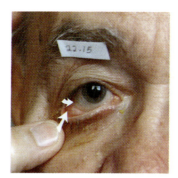

Figure 1.13b. Lower lid is everted with pressure applied to the lateral fatty area in the lid to herniate the fat at the lower tarsal plate—large arrow. Small arrow denotes area of scleral insertion of lateral rectus muscle.

Figure 1.14. (an overlay over Figure 1-27) Coronal section perpendicular to the optic nerve 9.4 mm anteriorly to the hind surface of the eye. *: connective tissue septa, atc: adipose tissue compartment. Arrows point to the ATCs. (With permission from Swets & Zeitlinger BV)

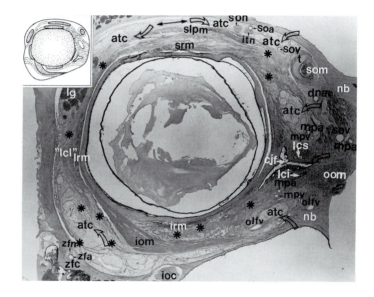

followed into the mid-orbit and then into the posterior orbit in subsequent sections of this chapter.

Branches of the infraorbital and zygomatic nerve to the lids and conjunctiva can be blocked preseptally by spread and diffusion from this 8:00 locus.

The site at 10:45 in the parasagittal plane of the lateral limbus clears the lacrimal gland and safely avoids the lacrimal or frontal nerves or the superior rectus/levator complex. Anesthetic injected preseptally from this locus infiltrates the upper lid to block orbicularis and sensory branches of the upper lid laterally, as does anesthetic injected at the 3:00 to 4:00 site when injection is made anterior to the medial canthal tendon and hydraulically enters the preseptal space.

Bulbar chemosis, often seen with "periocular blocks" or transconjunctival blocks done through the conjunctival sulcus, can be minimized by entering the anterior orbit between the anterior and posterior lamellae of the capsulopalpebral fascia or between the anterior lamella and the periorbit, not between the sclera and the anterior lamella, Figure 1.15 (see also Figure 1.34). Chemosis produced by percutaneous injection in the orbit suggests that the needle track was between the globe and the posterior lamella of the capsulopalpebral fascia. Transconjunctival injection through the palpebral fornix induces chemosis because it frequently makes a track between the globe and the posterior lamella.

Anesthetics injected in the anterior orbit diffuse through adipose compartments and through herniations in the orbital septum to block the orbicularis muscle. Therefore, a separate block of the facial nerve or its branches is necessary only when the orbital septum is unusually well developed, when block of the extraorbital facial musculature is desired, when a prolonged lid block is desired, or for the occasional patient with very small tense lids. Extraorbital block of the facial nerve is presented exceptionally well by Zahl.[65]

Spatial Relationships of the Globe and Orbit—the Mid-Orbit

A needle entering the orbit from any percutaneous or transconjunctival site approaches the plane of the equator of the eye in 2 to 4 mm in forward eyes (see Figure 1.7b) and in 5 to 10 mm in deep set eyes (shown in Figure 1.8b). When the needle point approaches the equator of the globe, it is well into the mid-orbit.

The mid-orbit begins anteriorly when the septal attachments of the extraocular muscles attach to the periorbit or globe and ends posteriorly about 10 to 12 mm from the hind surface of the globe where the bellies of the extraocular muscles are very large in comparison to the adipose tissue between them. The mid-orbit, therefore, is a space starting 10 to 15 mm anterior to the hind surface of the eye and ending 10 to 12 mm posterior to the hind surface of the eye—a distance that will average 25 mm. However, it may be as short as 12 mm in some people and as long as 35 mm in others, depending upon the length and position of the globe.

Geometric Considerations and Orbital Volume

The average globe is roughly 25 mm long from the front of the cornea to the back of the sclera; however, 20 and 30 mm globes are not rare. The axial length of the eye obtained by ultrasound is from the front of the cornea to the macula, which averages 23 mm (Figure 1.16). It is approximately 25 mm from the hind surface of the eye to the orbital apex, but 15 mm is not rare. Averages are depicted in Figure 1.16. Variation can be appreciated by studying Figures 1.51 b & c.

Figure 1.16 shows the geometric relationship in the transverse plane of the orbit, the globe, and the optic canal (shown in Figures 1.2 and 1.25 for schematic of the planes of the orbit).

When a needle is placed tangent to the globe at the equator medially from 2:30 to 3:00 parallel to the optical axis, i.e. in the sagittal and transverse planes, it directly enters the optic canal. The distance is much less than the needle must travel if it is introduced as a tangent at the lateral inferior orbital rim because of the 45 degree relationship between the lateral orbital wall and sagittal plane. The 45 degree relationship of the lateral orbital wall and the medial position of the optic canal must be remembered as needles are introduced into the orbit. The orbital apex is medial to the globe and not behind it, in contrast to its appearance in many artist's drawings made from the orbital axis projection.

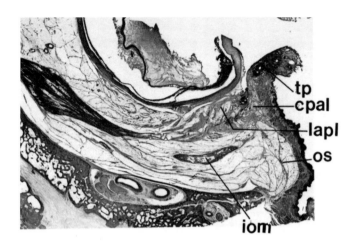

Figure 1.15. Magnification of an area of the mid-sagittal section of the inferior lid to show the connective tissue between the inferior rectus muscle, the lower eyelid, and the periorbit. This section is approximately the mid-sagittal plane of the globe parallel to the optic nerve. Note the space between the inferior oblique and inferior rectus muscles and the layers of the lids with the eye closed. The conjunctival fornix leads to a space between the posterior lamella of the capsulopalpebral ligament and Tenon's capsule; a needle taking this path into the space posterior to Tenon's will readily cause bulbar chemosis, whereas, percutaneous or transconjunctival injection just at the edge of the tarsal plate in the retracted lid will go anterior to the anterior lamella and will rarely dissect a path to the bulbar conjunctiva. A needle path lateral to the lateral limbus will avoid the inferior rectus and inferior oblique muscles. (With permission from Professional & Scientific Publishers)

The length of the orbital walls and the distance from the equator to the orbital apex are the primary determinants of orbital volume, which can vary from 8 to 30 ml.[20] To date, there are no good studies relating the volume of the orbit to the efficiency of blocking. It is likely that the smaller the volume of the orbit, the higher the concentration of local anesthetic, and therefore the more efficient the block. However, the septa of small orbits can be non-compliant and restrict flow of anesthetic from injection site to sensory nerves or branches of the oculomotor nerve.

A small orbital opening does not mean that the volume of the orbit will be small. The concavities of the orbit posterior to the opening can be extensive. A small orbital opening can be deceptive and mask a deep set globe with a large orbital depth and a resultant high orbital volume.

The greater the orbital volume (lengths of the medial and lateral orbital walls) the less likelihood that a good block will result from a small volume of anesthetic due to the greater orbital volume and longer distance to the sensory nerves or the oculomotor nerve. However, the volume of the orbit or the distance to the cone is rarely known before injecting local anesthetics. Someday this information may be as accessible to clinicians as the axial length of the globe is today, but not until theoretical and technical problems are solved.[21] Until then depth can only be inferred from the anesthetic effect of a given volume of anesthetic solution and the compliance of the orbit; the latter can be very deceiving.

The structures in the apex of the small orbit will be injured inadvertently by needles of average length (Figure 1.17). Katsev et al have discussed needle path length, orbital length, and the risk of injury from needles.[22] Figure 1.17 b & c show the distance, average and range, measured in 60 skulls by their method[22] and relate their data to the skull featured in Figure 1.2.

Katsev et al suggest that those doing "retrobulbar blocks" recognize that the use of a needle more than 31 mm may damage the optic nerve or structures in the orbital apex. They believe that needles 32 mm (1.25″) or larger should not be used and we agree.

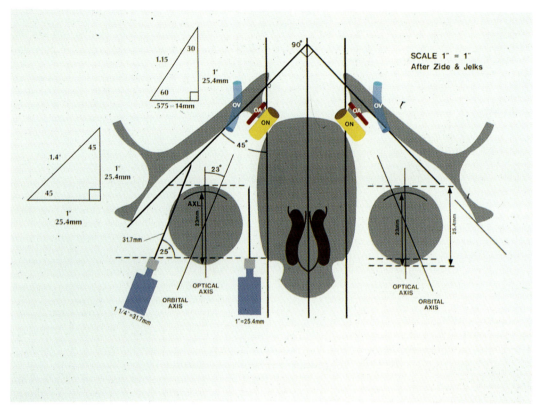

Figure 1.16. Schematic showing the geometric relationship of the walls of the orbit. This is a transverse section of average anatomic dimension in the transverse plane through the center of the pupil. The diagram is in anatomic size. The globe is 25 mm in length, and the distance from the hind surface of the eye to the orbital apex is 25 mm in length; these are averages. The optic nerve does not lie in the orbital apex, but the ophthalmic artery does. The superior ophthalmic vein is lateral and superior.

The plane of the iris makes a good measuring tool to determine the length to which needles have been introduced into the orbit. The optical axis, sighting down the center of the pupil when a patient is looking straight ahead makes an excellent reference to where structures will be in the sagittal plane. In this figure two needles are placed: (1) a 25 mm needle in the medial compartment in the transverse plane with the hub of the needle intersecting the plane of the iris; (2) a 31.7 mm needle in the transverse plane lateral to the lateral limbus beneath the globe just superior to the inferior orbital ridge. This plane is 8 mm inferior to the transverse plane.

When a 31.7 mm needle is inserted at the infero-temporal quadrant parallel to the orbital axis, and its hub intersects the plane of the iris in a globe of 25.4 mm length, the point of the needle is 3 to 5 mm from the hind surface of the eye. The needle would have passed through the equator of the eye if it were not 5 mm below the equator in the plane of the inferior limbus.

However, the optic nerve can be encountered at less than 20 mm in the mid-orbit when needles are inserted and aimed at the orbital apex using the principles of "Atkinson technique"[23,24] in forward eyes and changing the angles only slightly.

Blocks performed from the nasal aspect of the orbit must be done with needles

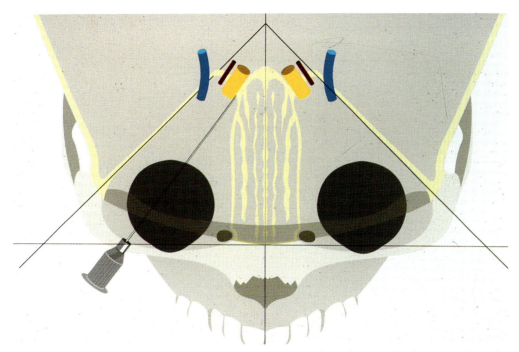

Figure 1.17a. A computer-generated drawing through the inferior orbital rim to show the orbital path length at the plane of the infero-temporal limbus to correspond to "retrobulbar needle path length" of Katsev et al. The study of Katsev et al defined retrobulbar needle path length as "the distance from the superior edge of the inferior temporal orbital rim to the superior nasal edge of the optic foramen."[22]

Because of tilting, this edge of the optic foramen is more anterior and the needle path length shorter, but this is how the needle could be directed to perforate the optic nerve. The measurement is easy to obtain in skulls .

shorter than 31 mm or injury can occur to the medial rectus muscle and the optic nerve. In fact, if 31 mm needles are used in the nasal hemisphere, the hub of the needle must never be inserted past the frontal plane of the limbus for risk of the needle entering orbital apex structures. The cone can be entered easily from the superior nasal quadrant with a 15 mm needle and the optic nerve speared in the orbital apex with a 31 mm needle in small orbits, if the needle hub pushes the upper lid to its concave maximum. The efficacy of "posterior peribulbar blocks" is partly due to the ease of intraconal injection of anesthetic in this quadrant by this mechanism.

Figure 1.16 shows the approximate relationship of globe length to needles being used. The geometric relationship between the hub of the needle and the point of the needle is evident. Needles introduced in the sagittal plane travel a greater distance toward the optic nerve than do needles introduced laterally along the orbital wall.

When the length of the globe is known, as it should be in modern ophthalmic clinics, geometry can be used to judge reasonably accurately the distance of the needle from the hind surface of the eye (as seen in Figure 1.59). A clear visualization of the position of the needle point should be made with reference to the globe instead of, or in addition to, bony landmarks because of the variations in orbital size, globe size, and depth of the globe in the

Figure 1.17b. A plot of the data obtained by Katsev et al as to the retrobulbar needle path length versus the frequency with which it was seen in 60 skulls. Note the skull and the computer generated images used in this book are at the approximate mean of their data. There was wide variation in retrobulbar needle path length. The shortest in the group of 120 orbits was 42 mm. Their data are similar to data of 1933 by Gifford[33] and 1972 by Linn and Smith.[47a] All three authors are concerned about damage to the optic nerve where it becomes fixed as it approaches the orbital apex to enter the optic canal.

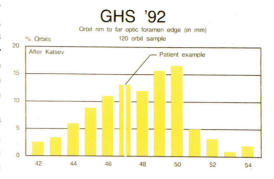

Figure 1.17c. Katsev et al subtracted the distance of the ciliary ganglion to the apex of the orbit (7 mm) and subtracted that from path length to generate a plot of relative risk of damage to the "fixed optic" nerve. Their data suggest that needles longer than 31.7 mm have significant risk of damage in short orbits. However, damage to the central retinal artery can occur 15 mm before the orbital apex. Therefore, in shallow orbits even the 31.7 mm needle needs to be used with caution .

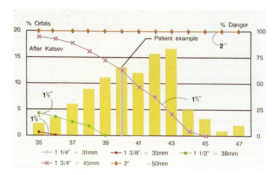

orbit. The plane of the iris (plane of the limbus) and the center of the pupil in forward gaze are meaningful reference points.

Just as it is important that needles do not enter the orbital apex because the orbit is too short (or the needle too long), it is imperative that needles do not penetrate the globe because the person administering the anesthetic block is unaware of the position of the equator or of the posterior hemisphere of the globe.

Perforation of the globe anterior to the equator has occurred during lid blocks when the lids are closed or during eye blocks when the relationship of the equator of the eye to the diameter of the globe is not considered. This is less likely to happen if the lids are open to expose the globe when a needle enters the orbit.

There is a positive relationship between the axial length of the eye and the diameter of the equator of the eye, although most large myopic eyes tend to be longer than they are in frontal diameter and therefore perforation is more likely in the posterior quadrant using "Atkinson technique".[23,24] Nonetheless, most myopic globes have a greater equatorial diameter and the sclera is thinner and anterior perforation more likely by the inexperienced blocker.

Many injuries to the globe behind the equator have occurred by having myopic patients look away from the needle.[25] In such patients with an elongated globe, the globe moves about an imaginary point through its central axis, placing the posterior pole (and the optic nerve) more in the path of the needle. The same phenomenon occurs when digital pressure is applied to the globe anterior to the equator to push it out of the needle path; the posterior globe can be rotated into the needle path by this maneuver.

Unsold,[26] Pautler,[25] and Grizzard[27] believe that having the patient look superonasally should be abandoned for retrobulbar blocks done from the inferotemporal compartment because the optic nerve is placed more in the path of the needle and is made more taut (Figure 1.18 a & b).

It can be frightening to some patients to look straight ahead or towards the needle when injections are made in the orbit, however, anatomically this is much safer. Figures 1.18 a & b and 1.19 show the relationship of the "up-and-in" eye position to needles entering the optic nerve which is stretched when the patient looks away from the needle; it is easier for needles to perforate the nerve in this position because of displacement and stretch.[25,27] Damage to the optic nerve or subarachnoid injection of anesthetic in the nerve sheath can more readily occur.

However, little attention has been paid to the danger of having patients look away from the needle point or danger of pushing the globe away from the needle in peribulbar blocks. The posterior globe is not necessarily moved away from the needle by pushing on the anterior globe, but can be placed more in the needle path by this maneuver.

Fear induced by the patient seeing the needle can be eliminated by standing at the

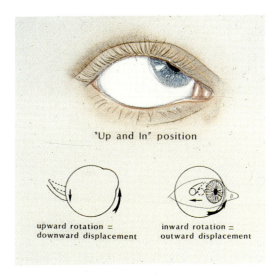

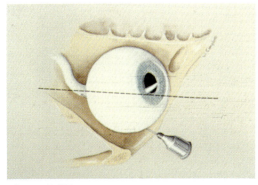

Figure 1.18b.

Figure 1.18a & b. The "up and in" position of the eye causes (a) downward and (b) outward displacement of the optic nerve into the path of the retrobulbar needle. (Courtesy of Scott Pautler, MD, Tampa, Florida)

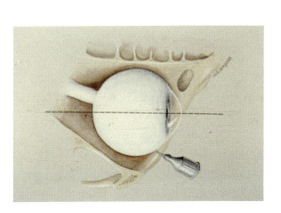

Figure 1.19. With the patient's eyes in the primary gaze, a sharp, 3.2-cm (1 1/4"), 27-gauge needle is introduced through the skin, above the inferior orbital rim, between the temporal limbus and the lateral canthus. The needle is directed toward an imaginary area behind the macula to avoid crossing a sagittal plane through the visual axis. (Courtesy of Scott Pautler, MD, Tampa, Florida)

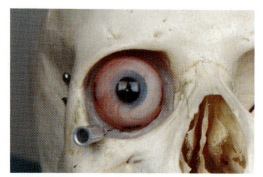

Figure 1.20a.

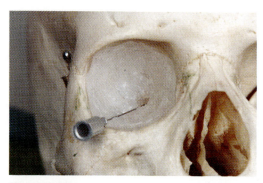

Figure 1.20b.

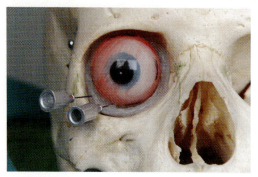

Figure 1.20c.

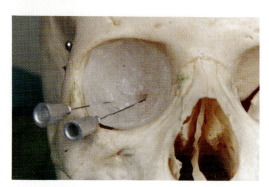

Figure 1.20d.

Figure 1.20. The skull of Figure 1.1 with a 25-mm (1″) artificial eye with the insertions of the rectus muscles painted on it in black seated on a matrix of silicon. Note the needle paths and the proximity of the needles to the equator of the eye when the globe is removed. (a) A 1 1/4″ needle is inserted according to Atkinson technique. (b) "a" with globe removed (c) A 1-1/4″ needle inserted at the 8:00 position at a 30 degree angle to the optical axis. Note the extra space and how clear the needle is of the optic nerve. (d) "c" with globe removed (e) needles inserted for the medial block at 4:00 and for a supero-temporal block at 10:45. (f) "e" with globe removed (g) shows the relation of the globe, needles, and equator in the sagittal plane. (h) Frontal histological sections of the orbit can be stacked between layers of the silicone and placed in the orbit, so that relations can be better appreciated. A color contact print of a histologic section cut perpendicular to the optic nerve at 5 mm behind the eye (Figure 1.31) has been cut out along the bone edge and placed in the orbit to show the anatomy at 5 mm behind the hind surface of the globe.

patient's side out of his or her peripheral vision and having the patient look straight ahead at a suitable object.

Anatomical insight and adequate surgical exposure prevent injury. When the eye is open so that the slightest motion can be a sign of contact with a septum, a muscle, or the sclera, then injury or perforation is extremely unlikely.

Methods to Study the Anatomy of the Mid-Orbit

The relationship of needle path to orbital structures beyond the equator cannot be studied well by dissection; it is necessary to study orbital sections of fixed cadavers.

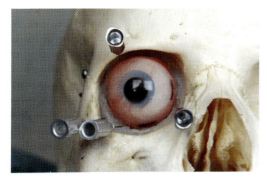

Figure 1.20e.

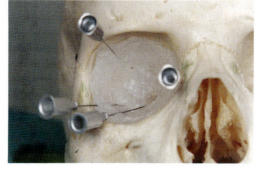

Figure 1.20f.

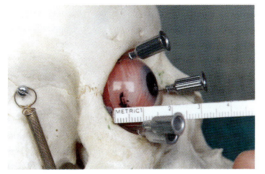

Figure 1.20g.

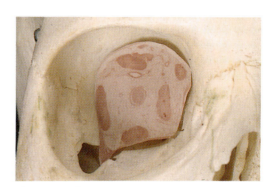

Figure 1.20h.

Unfortunately rigor mortis changes slightly the position of the globe within the orbit. During death, ocular muscles tend to withdraw the globe slightly into the orbit so measurements from the apex of the orbit to the equator of the globe in fixed specimens are slightly less than the exact distances in life.

These differences in the depth of the mid-orbit are relatively insignificant in performing blocks in cadaver eyes in training but need to be considered. Practice on formalin-fixed or cold fresh cadaver orbits sounds like a good solution to practicing blocks, but in addition to the slight change of depth, there is the dissimilar resiliency of cadaver tissues. The soft "feel" of the adipose tissue compartments is changed by fixation.

One should study the human skull and place a suitable model eye into the orbit before making injections in the orbit (Figure 20a-h) (also shown in Figure 1.1). A 25 mm globe was placed in the skull in Figure 1.20 and the globe is supported on a silicone matrix which can be changed to duplicate deep and shallow globe position. Needles can be inserted into the silicone and proximity to the skull and optic nerve recognized.

Koornneef's sections (shown in Figures 1.26 through 1.40) can be appropriately reduced in size or those of Figures 1.41 through 1.52 can be cut out and placed in proper perspective within the orbit behind the model globe as in Figure 1.20h. (Remember Koornneef's frontal sections are cut perpendicular to the optic nerve (Figure 1.21), except for Figure 1.29 and 1.34 , or about 25 degrees off the true frontal plane.)

A needle passing the equator inclined 10 degrees toward the optical axis from any "periocular or peribulbar site" will be in one of the rectus muscles or between two of them.

The muscles hardly move during the various positions of gaze because of their attachments by the septa to the periorbit and to the optic nerve,[28] so going between them is the first necessary skill in planning an approach to the mid-orbit.

The muscle cone is not presented to the needle by having the patient look up and nasal as many books teach. Going through the muscles with a needle or injecting local anesthetic into them has a high risk of inducing myotoxic, neurologic, or fibrotic changes.[29-31]

Injection of dyes in the orbit to outline the tracks of needles is of limited value as a learning tool because the dyes disperse so quickly within the orbit that it makes needle pathway difficult to visualize, however, the exercise is most valuable (Figure 1.22). The ready movement of dyes in the orbit in most specimens is one reason that the globe was thought to float in a sea of fat lobules instead of being separated into compartments by the septa. Injection of thin latex material followed by clearing of the specimen gives an idea of track and bulk flow of aqueous solution. Figure 1.23 shows the distribution of the injectate into the orbit and lids from an "Atkinson" conal injection site.

Figure 1.24 shows an orbital cadaver dissection in which the arteries have been filled with red latex.

Histologic section analysis will elucidate better needle pathways into the orbit, present anatomical detail, and show the relationship of the mid- and posterior orbit.

The orbits were sectioned as per Figure 1.25. Note that the frontal (coronal) and sagittal sections orient to the orbital axis of the anatomist except for Figures 1.29 and 1.34, which are true frontal sections.

Figures 1.26 through 1.35 are "frontal sections" approximately 3 to 5 mm apart from the front of the eye to the apex of the orbit. The specimens were sectioned perpendicular to the optic nerve or in the orbital axis—20 to 25 degrees from a true frontal plane, as anatomists ordinarily are interested in the relationship of structures to the optic nerve. Figures 1.29 and 1.34 are thick cleared sections cut in the true frontal plane.

The insert in the left upper portion of sections shows the location of the septa at that level.

Figure 1.26 is at the equator of the globe or 12 mm anterior to the hind surface. Figure 1.27 is 3 mm posterior to the equator or 10 mm anterior to the hind surface. Figure 1.28 is 7 mm posterior to the equator or 5 mm anterior to the hind surface. Figure 1.29 is a thick true frontal section at approximately 6 mm from the hind surface. Figure 1.30 is 12 mm posterior to the equator or at the hind surface. Figure 1.31 is 5 mm posterior to the hind surface, Figure 1.32 is 10 mm posterior to the hind surface, Figure 1.33 is 15 mm posterior, Figure 1.34 is a true coronal thick section 15 mm behind the eye and Figure 1.35 is 20 mm posterior to the hind surface of the globe or deep in the apex.

Note that at 10 mm behind the hind surface the rectus muscles begin to converge. At 15 mm behind the hind surface there is little space between the muscles; the muscles form a "muscular cone." The arteries, veins, and nerves are compressed against one another and are vulnerable targets for needles. The posterior orbit is entered when the fat between the muscles is small in comparison to the size of the muscle belly. Sections in Figures 1.33, 1.34 and 1.35 are located in posterior orbit.

The mid-transverse and mid-sagittal sections extend from the anterior to the posterior orbit. The transverse sections of the orbit start with Figure 1.36. The first section is in the superior part of the orbit through the trochlea. Note how easily the trochlea and the superior ophthalmic vein can be injured by needle passage through the superior nasal quadrant. Many structures are easily injured in the superior nasal compartment when a needle enters it directly through the skin (see also Figure 1.3).

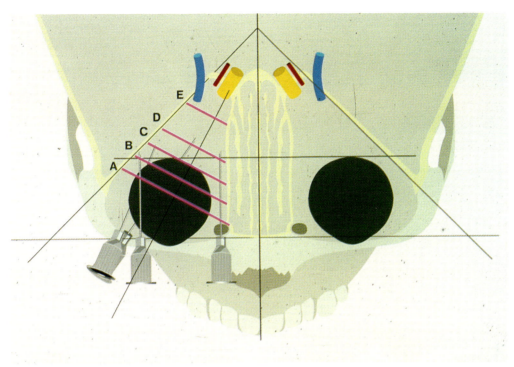

Figure 1.21. A computer-generated transverse image of the results of Figure 1.20 showing the approximate points of the needles when inserted as above. The planes A, B, C, D, and E perpendicular to the orbital axis are the planes of the histologic sections (Figures 1.29-1.35). Most orbital anatomy coronal sections of the orbit were done perpendicular to the optic nerve as were most of the CT scans until recently. True coronal sections are Figures 1.29, 1.34, and 1.41-1.52 .

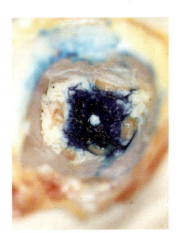

Figure 1.22. A 27 gauge 1 1/4" needle was introduced at 4:00 into the left orbit of a refrigerated fresh cadaver and 0.5 ml of methylene blue solution was injected as the needle was withdrawn. The orbit was then transected by a very sharp knife 5 mm behind the hind surface of the globe. Note how the dye has distributed throughout most of the orbit. Neither the needle track nor the point of injection can be deduced. (Courtesy of RC Hamilton, MB, BCh)

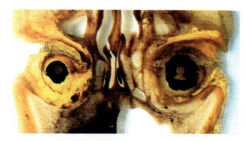

Figure 1.23a.

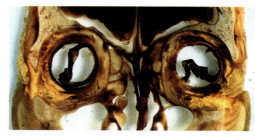

Figure 1.23b.

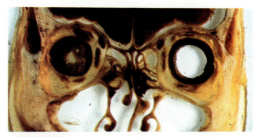

Figure 1.23c.

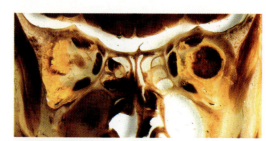

Figure 1.23d.

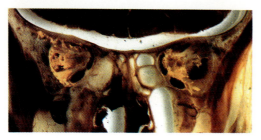

Figure 1.23e.

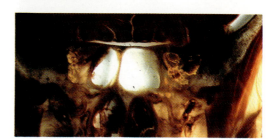

Figure 1.23f.

Figure 1.23a-f. Synthetic rubber compound, 4 ml injected into each orbit according to the Atkinson technique and the specimen cleared and sectioned frontally in 5-mm slices. Note the injected compound fills the orbit and the lids on both sides. Some small amount follows the optic chiasm and along the left optic nerve. This optic sheath dural attachment to the skull must have been hydraulically perforated during injection; similar perforation was shown in CT scan by Zahl with 8 ml peribulbar injection.[67]

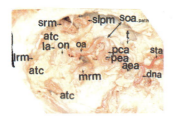

Figure 1.24. An orbital cadaver dissection in which the arterial system was injected with red latex at the time of preparation of the cadaver. Dissection shows how the posterior orbit is filled with blood vessels and how tortuous the arteries can be in the superior nasal quadrant of the elderly. (Courtesy G. Fanning, MD)

Figure 1.25. Drawings showing the planes along which the orbits were sectioned histologically and by computed tomography (CT). True frontal or coronal; Frontal or coronal perpendicular to the optic nerve; Transverse; Sagittal parallel to the optic nerve which is approximately parallel to the orbital axis; True sagittal. See Figure 1.21 for transverse plane and Figure 1.1 for further orientation.

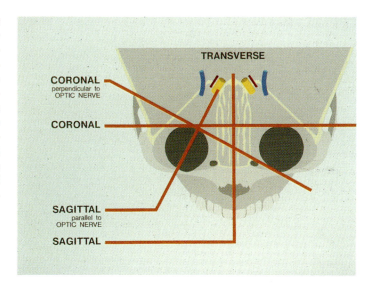

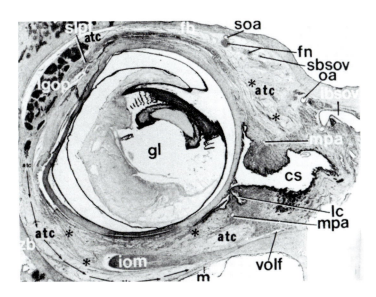

Figure 1.26. A coronal section cut perpendicular to the optic nerve or approximately in the orbital axis. About 12.4 mm anterior to the hind surface of the globe. Note the section goes between the lacrimal gland temporally and conjunctival fornix medially. It shows the origin of the inferior oblique muscle and fibers of Tenon's capsule overlying the superior and inferior rectus muscles. The adipose tissue compartments at 1:30, 3:00, 4:00, and 6:30-8:00 are evident. (With permission from MP Bergen, MD and Swets & Zeitlinger BV)

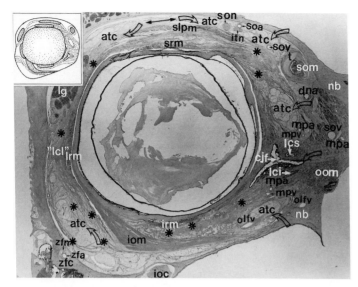

Figure 1.27. A coronal section cut perpendicular to the optic nerve or approximately in the orbital axis, about 10.5 mm anterior to the hind surface of the globe. Temporally the lacrimal gland is a bit smaller and an adipose tissue compartment appears at 10:45. The trochlea is present medially as well as the adipose tissue compartments above and below it. The conjunctival fornix in the area of the canthal tendon is adjacent to it nasally. The adipose tissue compartment between 6:30 and 8:00 is quite in evidence. Note the inferior oblique muscle is now sliding alongside the globe and there are fibers of the lateral, superior, and inferior rectus muscles attached to Tenon's. (With permission from Swets & Zeitlinger BV)

Figure 1.28. A coronal section parallel to the orbital axis 4.6 mm anterior to the hind surface of the globe. Notice that the medial rectus muscle is firmly attached to the globe, but there is connective tissue between the other three and the globe. The ATCs are well defined, especially at 7:00-8:00. The ATC between 1:30 and 2:30 is now beginning to fill with arteries, veins, and nerves. The ATC to the medial caruncle is now obvious as are fibers of the orbicularis muscle overlying it. Notice a number of venous channels in the 4:30 ATC, and that there is only a small amount of space between the inferior rectus muscle and its underlying maxillary sinus. Notice the openness of the 7:30-8:00 ATC. Adjacent temporally to the inferior rectus muscle are the artery and nerve to the inferior oblique muscle, above the orbital floor just temporal to the muscle where they could easily be injured by an orbital floor approach. (With permission from Swets & Zeitlinger BV)

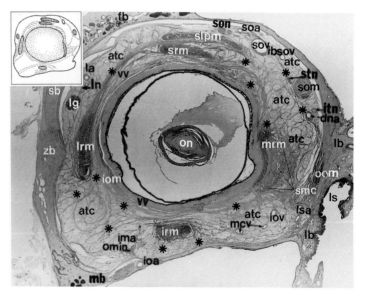

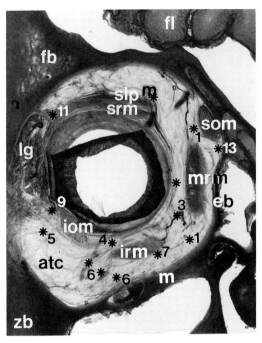

Figure 1.29. A .5 cm coronal histologic section of the right orbit which had been stained then cleared to demonstrate the A-P continuity of the septa, approximately 5 mm anterior to the hind surface of the globe. The section, viewed with a binocular microscope shows that the septa go in an anterior-posterior direction and have considerable thickness. The major septa 5 mm anterior to the hind portion of the globe are marked, highlighted, and numbered according to the numbering system in the table of abbreviations.

Notice the septa of the medial rectus muscle going to the roof and floor of the orbit and the septum which runs from it to the inferior rectus muscle. The superior rectus muscle has attachments to the floor of the orbit, to the inferior oblique muscle and to the lateral rectus muscle. These septal attachments are very close to the globe. A supero-nasal needle tra-jectory taking it through the septa will put it in intimate contact with the optic nerve at about 10 mm from the hind surface of the globe.

The ATC between the inferior oblique muscle and the orbital wall minor septa going to it. There is a large septum at 10:30 joining the superior levator to the lateral rectus muscle and an ATC above and nasal to it.

The section is at approximately the same level as Figure 1.28, but cut in the "true" coronal plane. Note that the globe in this specimen is much more anterior than the globe in specimen 1.28. In 1.28 the lacrimal sac is present, whereas in 1.29 the lacrimal sac is anterior. (With permission from Blackwell Scientific Publications)

Access to the superior nasal adipose compartment to block the superior rectus, levator, superior oblique muscle, and the frontal nerve is somewhat safer through the infratrochlear approach and much safer through the medial canthal approach to avoid the trochlea and vascular structures of the superonasal area.

Figure 1.37 is a mid-transverse section through the center of the lens of the eye. Notice the degree of curvature of the path of the optic nerve and lateral rectus muscle. Figure 1.38 is through the inferior limbus from 4:00 to 8:00 to show the ATCs.

Figures 1.39 and 1.40 are sagittal sections cut parallel to the optic nerve rather than true sagittal sections; they follow the orbital axis. Figure 1.39 is mid-sagittal through the lens. Figure 1.40 is at the lateral limbus; note the superior and infero-temporal adipose compartments. A needle would traverse this plane if inserted at the lateral limbus in a plane parallel to the optic nerve. It would reach the lateral wall of the orbit, not the orbital apex if inserted in the optical axis.

Figures 1.41 through 1.52 correlate Figures 1.26 through 1.40 with CT sections and cryosections from similar areas; the "a" and "b" are CT scans and cryosections which are true frontal (coronal) or true sagittal as are Figures 1.29 and 1.34. Note in Figure 1.42 the difference in fat-filled space between the equator of the eye and the bones in the two specimens. This is patient variation, not preparation of specimens; some people have little fat around the globe at the equator. Note how small the orbital apex is in Figure 1.47. Is

Figure 1.30. A coronal section parallel to the orbital axis through the hind surface of the globe passing through the posterior surface of Tenon's capsule. Notice the ciliary arteries entering the globe and note the subarachnoid space between the dura and the optic nerve. The ATC at 1:00 is now filled with blood vessels. The superior ophthalmic vein is beginning to move obliquely across the orbit, and will travel nasal to temporal in about a 45 degree angle. Notice the veins, arteries, and nerves in the supero-nasal quadrant. The ATC at 2:30 appears to be quite open for injection, however, re-

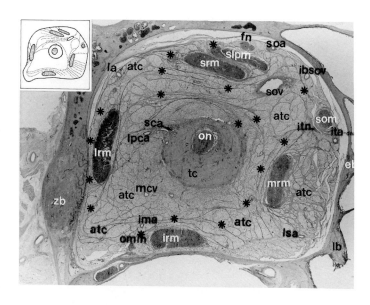

member the trochlear tendon would have just crossed it anteriorly.

The ATC between the medial rectus muscle and the nasal and ethmoid bones is quite obvious as well as its communication with the 2:30 ATC and the 4:30 ATC. Anesthetic placed in this "medial pericone compartment" will spread in all directions to usually block the motor nerve to the superior oblique muscle, to the superior rectus muscle, to the levator muscle, will usually block the supratrochlear nerve, the supraorbital nerve, the infratrochlear nerve, and the nerve to the lacrimal sack. The ATC between 6:30 and 8:00 is quite evident as well as the cellules of adipose tissue in it.

At this level there appears to be a central adipose compartment of sorts surrounding the optic nerve containing the ciliary nerves. Anesthetics injected in this central space would tend to travel centrally. This may lead to an increased effectiveness of sub-Tenon's injected anesthetics injected through Tenon's into the retrobulbar space.

Note how the inferior rectus muscle and the lateral rectus muscle are already quite adherent to bone. Notice the inferior muscular artery and the oculomotor nerve to the inferior oblique muscle temporal to the inferior rectus muscle. The ATC at 7:30 to 8:00 is quite wide open for placing anesthetics in a relatively avascular place; however, it is separated into peripheral and central sub-compartments. (With permission from Swets & Zeitlinger)

it advisable to place a sharp needle deep into the cone just to get a faster block or use a bit less anesthetic?

In real life the size and paths of the avascular tunnels are hidden by skin or conjunctiva, as is the space between the bone and the globe. Needles pass from anterior to posterior safely when the anatomy of these areas and the skill of locating them atraumatically are known (Figures 1.41 - 1.52).

The Five Safe Passageways

The histologic sections demonstrate the safe areas through which needles may be passed to avoid the extraocular muscles, arteries, veins, and nerves. There are five such areas.

Four are located between the muscles and a fifth passage is nasal to the medial

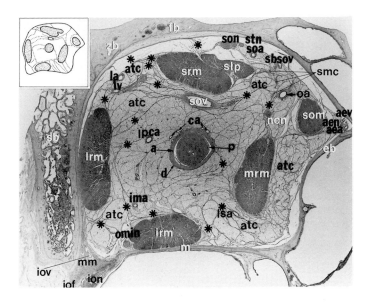

Figure 1.31. A coronal section perpendicular to the optic nerve 5.0 mm posterior to the hind surface of the globe. Note the nerves, arteries, and veins in the 1:30 to 2:30 ATC. A fairly thick septum exists now between the medial rectus muscle and the roof of the orbit. The inferior rectus and lateral rectus muscle are quite adherent to bone. The space between the inferior rectus muscle and the lateral rectus muscle is smaller. The central adipose compartment surrounding the optic nerve seems to be divided into superior and inferior hemispheres by the adipose tissue septum between the lateral rectus muscle and the optic nerve and the medial rectus muscle and the optic nerve. The superior ophthalmic vein is now directly above the optic nerve on its course laterally.

Note the thick septum supero-temporally between the lateral rectus muscle and the superior rectus muscle. The ATC lateral to that septum is now very small; however, going through that septum would gain access to the central compartment. (With permission from Swets & Zeitlinger BV)

rectus muscle. These areas roughly correspond to the adipose tissue compartments (abbreviated ATC in frontal sections). An ATC is a compartment of fatty tissues devoid of significant structures, making it an ideal conduit for needles. The walls of the ATCs contain veins; the ciliary arteries pass through septal walls to run inside of central adipose compartments as they move anteriorly.

The infero-temporal ATC is the route used by Labat,[32] Lowenstein, Duverger, Atkinson,[23,24] Gifford,[33] Gills,[34,35] Grizzard,[27] and Hamilton.[36] Once through the skin and orbital septum, then no further significant septa should be felt until the posterior orbit. In older patients even the orbital septum is attenuated.

Injection in the preseptal space anterior to the orbital septum will anesthetize motor fibers to the orbicularis, and sensory fibers to the lower lateral lid and conjunctiva. The preseptal space of the lower lid is best delineated by the transconjunctival approach. Evert and retract the lower lid, then penetrate the orbital septum while injecting anesthetic. Anesthetic will diffuse preseptally to block orbicularis and lateral inferior sensory fibers to the bulbar conjunctiva and lids (as shown in Figures 1.7b and 1.13b).

The infero-temporal compartment blends into the muscular cone smoothly, almost continuously, because there is no major septum connecting the lateral rectus muscle to the inferior rectus muscle (see Figures 1.30 through 1.35). There are only minor septa, like layers of an onion, through which the needle should pass until the septum of the central compartment is reached.

Figure 1.32. A coronal section 9.5 mm posterior to the hind surface of the globe. Note the compactness of the structures. There is very little space between any of the rectus muscles; space superiorly is occupied by the ophthalmic artery nasally and the superior ophthalmic vein temporally. Notice, at this level, the trochlear nerve, the abducens nerve, and the oculomotor nerve are entering the muscle hila. Many of the branches of the ophthalmic artery have been cut in cross section at this level. The lacrimal artery, the posterior ciliary arteries, the ciliary ganglion, and the nasociliary nerve are probably sectioned.

Note the central retinal artery is in the optic nerve sheath and more anteriorly it will penetrate the optic nerve on the inferior surface. (With permission from Swets & Zeitlinger BV)

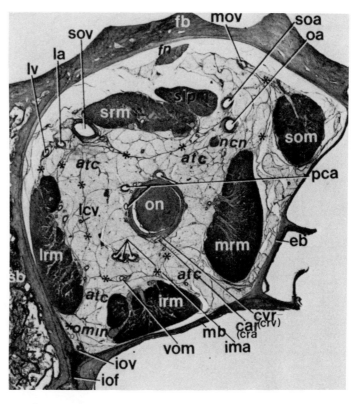

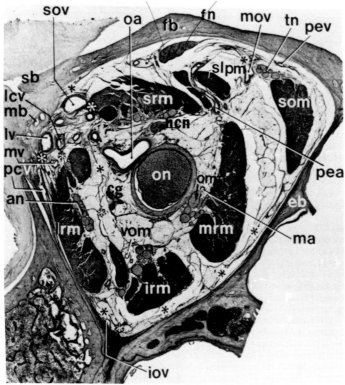

Figure 1.33. A coronal section perpendicular to the optic nerve 15.5 mm posterior to the hind surface of the globe. Septa divide it into superior and inferior compartments. The ophthalmic artery is cut where it branches into the lacrimal artery just as it starts to proceed over the top of the optic nerve. Note the branches of the oculomotor nerve, the trochlear nerve, and the abducens nerve are not covered by connective tissue before they move anteriorly to enter the hilum of the muscles. The nasociliary artery and the ciliary ganglion are quite obvious. Anesthetic placed in this area should cause profound nerve block since there is very little connective tissue separating anesthetic from the nerve, but the needles could injure or cut "fixed" structures. (With permission from Swets & Zeitlinger BV)

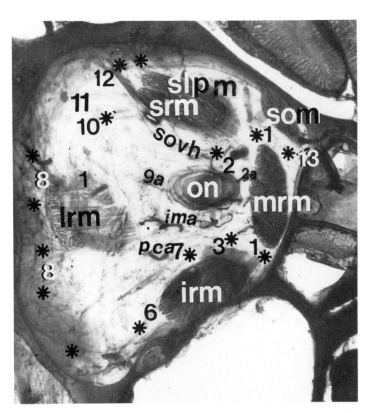

Figure 1.34. A true coronal histologic thick section (0.5 cm) at approximately 10 to 15 mm posterior to the hind surface of the globe which has been cleared to show the depth of the connective tissue. Note the septa between the optic nerve and the medial rectus muscle and between the optic nerve and the lateral rectus muscle. These septa are thick enough to dissuade perfusion between the infero-nasal compartment and the supero-nasal compartment which would, in this specimen, probably account for poor akinesia of the superior rectus, oblique and levator muscles from an inferior temporal injection. Notice the different perspective in the coronal plane—how close the optic nerve is to the medial wall of the orbit rather than being centered. While thick sections tend to show septal depth in the AP diameter, they lose much fine detail.

Numbers refer to septa found in the Table of Abbreviations. (With permission from Blackwell Scientific Publications)

The superior-temporal ATC is used by Knapp,[37] Braun,[38] Kelman,[39] and Thornton.[40] It is bounded by the periorbit and the septum connecting the lateral and superior rectus muscles to each other in the anterior and mid-orbit, but it opens into the cone in the posterior orbit. The connective tissue that connects the lateral rectus muscle to the superior rectus muscle anteriorly is dense fascia in most orbits (see Figures 1.27 and 1.28); penetrating or perforating it is palpable with a dull or sharp needle. Dull needles may hang up or flex during this penetration. It will be penetrated by a straight needle with 10 degree angulation to the optical axis, and it is penetrated easily by a bent needle, as described by Kelman[39] to provide an intraconal "retrobulbar block."

Penetrating this supero-temporal septum to provide access to the cone is more reliable at producing ocular akinesia than counting on anesthetic to follow fenestrations in the septa and enter the cone, as is done with lateral orbital blocks such as those described by Pitkin[41] and Adriani.[32] However, diffusion through thin septa or the posterior fenestration occurs because akinesia can be produced in some patients with the needle outside the septum deliberately hugging the orbit and not converged to the optical axis. The akinesia is often only partial from a single "periorbital injection" in this locus.

The superior orbital vein, located 10 to 15 mm from the hind surface of the eye, may be injured when injecting through the supero-temporal compartment, so the injection should be placed anterior to the vein (as shown in Figures 1.31 and 1.32). It is possible to

Figure 1.35. A coronal section perpendicular to the optic nerve 20.6 mm posterior to the hind surface of the globe. The muscles are blending into Zinn's annulus. Note the large size of the superior ophthalmic vein in comparison to the ophthalmic artery and all the important nerves entering the orbit. Obviously, needles should never be placed into this area or they will impinge some structure against bone. (With permission from Swets & Zeitlinger BV)

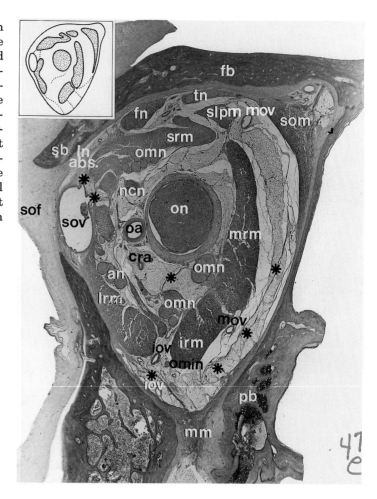

have vasomotor collapse from fast intravenous injection into the superior orbital vein. Deep injection could injure the nerves of the superior orbital fissure or penetrate the dura or cavernous sinus.

Injection in the supero-temporal compartment allows anesthetic easy access to the lacrimal and frontal nerves and provides conjunctival anesthesia, whereas the inferotemporal approach often misses these nerves. Bulk spread of anesthetic flows anterior to the overlying preseptal space, where it blocks the motor fibers to the orbicularis of the upper lid as well as sensory fibers to the upper lid temporally. However, the inferior orbicularis and sensory fibers to the lower lid and conjunctiva may be completely missed!

Preseptal injection of local in this compartment will block the orbicularis but often miss the sensory nerves to the bulbar conjunctiva and tarsus of the upper lid.

The medial ATC is extensive. It communicates with both the infero-nasal and supero-nasal ATCs. Each can be reached percutaneously, but both can be accessed from the medial canthal approach (as shown in Figures 1.28 through 1.31). These ATCs eventually communicate with the central oculomotor compartment throughout the mid-orbit and in the posterior orbit (see Figure 1.33).

A needle inserted through the medial palpebral fold (as shown in Figure 1.14)

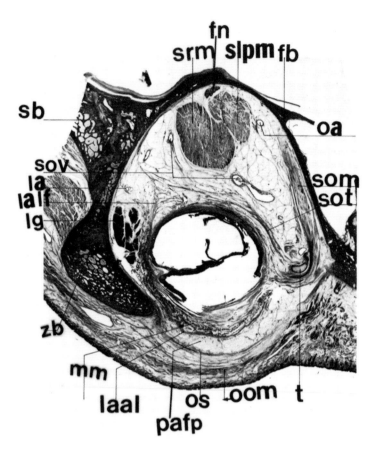

Figure 1.36. Transverse section through the upper one-third of the right orbit through the trochlea nasally and the lacrimal gland temporally. Both the supero-nasal and supero-temporal compartments appear relatively safe conduits for needles; however, the superior ophthalmic vein and ophthalmic artery are apparent in the superior nasal compartment. (With permission from Raven Press)

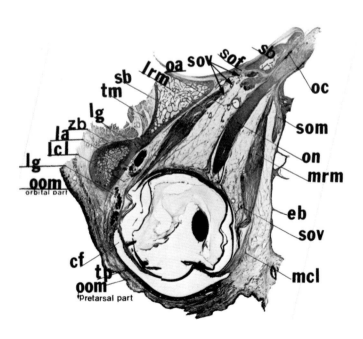

Figure 1.37. Transverse midaxial section through the optic nerve and the medial and lateral rectus muscles. The medial runs an A-P course, but the lateral is quite curved. Note that the diameter of the globe is roughly the distance from the hind surface of the eye to the apex. Notice the medial ATC between the medial rectus muscle and the medial orbital wall and connective tissue between the lateral rectus muscle and the lateral orbital wall.

A major septum runs from the hind surface of the eye between the optic nerve and the lateral rectus muscle, thus subdividing that space into central and lateral A-P compartments (Figure 1.55). (With permission from Raven Press)

Figure 1.38a. Transverse section below the optic nerve through both the medial and inferior rectus muscles. Note the medial ATC and its position to the medial rectus muscle. Note the septa running between the hind surface of the eye and the orbital apex subdividing that space into A-P compartments .

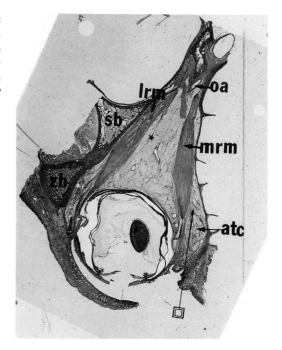

Figure 1.38b. 2 mm inferior to 1.38 a approximately at the inferior limbus. The lateral rectus muscle is still present and the inferior rectus is sectioned. The medial rectus muscle is no longer present posteriorly. Note the lateral ATC and the medial compartment which is full of veins. The septum dividing the lateral central compartment is still present and appears to connect with the inferior rectus muscle.

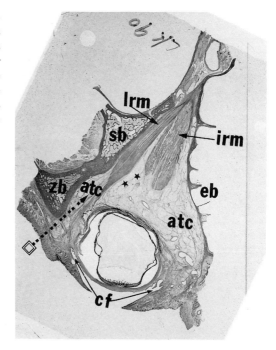

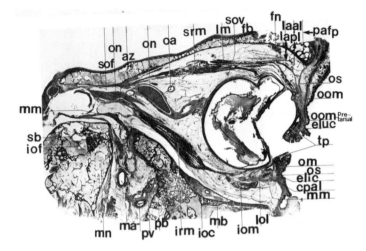

Figure 1.39. Mid-axial sagittal section through the center of the globe and the optic nerve. An artifact allows separation of the inferior rectus posteriorly from the bone. The superior and inferior ATCs septa sub-divide the central compartment superiorly. Note the frontal nerve adherent to the superior orbital periorbit. The space 10 mm behind the eye is crowded. Note the anterior and posterior lamellae of both the upper and lower lids and the relationship of the globe to the capsulo-palpebral fascia. (With permission from Raven Press)

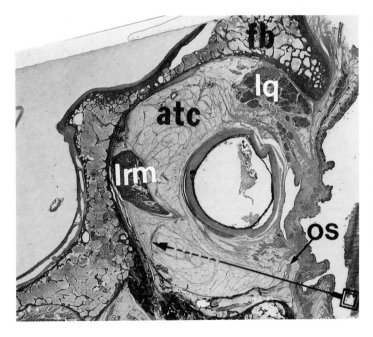

Figure 1.40. Sagittal section (parallel to the optic nerve plane) just lateral to the lateral limbus showing the inferior and superior ATCs. The lacrimal gland is present in this section showing that the section is somewhat lateral to the lateral limbus. Notice how totally undisturbed the infero-temporal ATC is when a needle goes parallel to the orbital axis. The needle would touch bone about 5 mm behind the hind surface of the eye if introduced in the optical axis or true sagittal plane.

tangential to the globe encounters the medial check ligament when directed 2 to 5 mm. At 1 to 2 mm more, it encounters the periosteum of the lacrimal bone allowing the operator to identify the medial orbital wall posterior to the posterior lacrimal crest.

If the needle point is retracted 2 mm and the angle of the shaft of the needle re-introduced in the sagittal plane or 5 degrees nasally, it will remain clear of the medial rectus muscle and travel down the medial compartment. However, it should never be inclined temporally between 2:00 to 4:00 or it may contact the medial rectus muscle, leading to hemorrhage or myotoxicity. The needle point should never pass

Figures c and d of 1.41 through 1.52 are shown in approximate anatomical size.

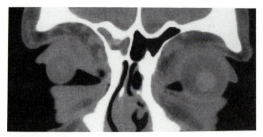

Figure 1.41a.

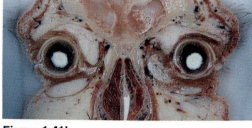

Figure 1.41b.

Figure 1.41. Frontal sections at the conjunctival sac area. Note the significant anatomical differences between the three presentations. In Figure 1.41b the conjunctival sac is present, and the globe is cut through the lens of the eye. The corresponding section, Figure 1.41c, shows the conjunctival sac area, but the globe is cut well behind the lens. The specimen that

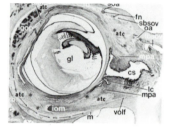

Figure 1.41c.

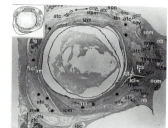

Figure 1.41d.

was cryosectioned, therefore has very deep set eyes. Note the amount of fat in the cryosection compared to the specimen in the histologic section—the cryosection specimen has much more orbital fat.

Orbits vary greatly in the amount of fat they contain, and this is a good example of those differences. At this level, the ATC has formed in 41c; it is larger in 41d. Note between 1:30 and 3:00 the number of structures that the needle would go through in the supero-nasal compartment.

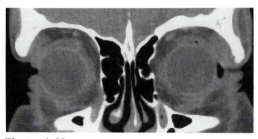

Figure 1.42a.

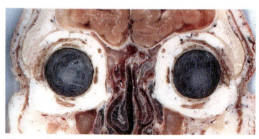

Figure 1.42b.

Figure 1.42. Frontal sections past the equator. The cryosection is from the same deep set eye of the preceding figure. The other sections are from eyes of normal depth. The infero-temporal fatty compartment is well developed as are the 10:30 and infero-nasal compartments. The medial compartment is very well developed and access to both the infero-nasal and

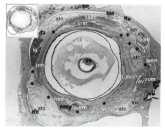

Figure 1.42c.

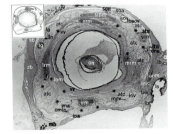

Figure 1.42d.

the supero-nasal compartments is quite clear of the medial rectus muscle.

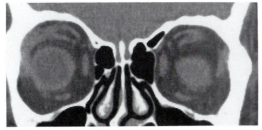

Figure 1.43a.

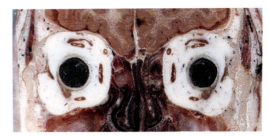

Figure 1.43b.

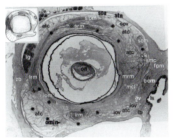

Figure 1.43c.

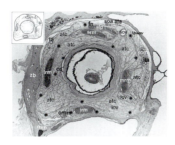

Figure 1.43d.

Figure 1.43. Frontal sections approximately 5 mm anterior to the hind surface of the eye. Note the inferior oblique muscle coursing onto the globe, and below it, the inferior rectus muscle. The inferior branch of the oculomotor nerve comes forward to innervate the inferior oblique muscle where it is readily injurable from blocks done in the classical position at the junction of the medial two-thirds and lateral one-third of the inferior orbital rim. The septa anchors the lateral rectus muscle to bone. The ATCs—medial, infero-temporal, and supero-temporal—are well defined and free of arteries or veins.   Medially there are fibers of the orbicularis oculi muscle; injections of local anesthetic in the medial compartment at this locus readily diffuse anteriorly to block the orbicularis the upper and lower lid. In Figure d, 2 mm deeper, orbicularis muscle is absent; the plane of diffusion to block the orbicularis is thus between c and d. The medial compartment is well defined, as is the access way superiorly 20 degrees and inferiorly to inject anesthetics more towards those quadrants. The infero-nasal, infero-temporal, and the supero-temporal ATCs are well developed. Note the thick connective tissue septum joining the superior rectus muscle and the lateral rectus muscle.

more than 2 mm posterior to the hind surface of the eye—a distance that can be calculated knowing the axial length (as shown in Figure 1.16). The needle can be inserted in the transverse plane of the orbit to enter the common medial ATC or inclined 10 degrees inferior or superior to the transverse plane to enter the adipose tissue compartments in the infero-nasal and superonasal areas.

Injection causes bulk posterior flow of anesthetic to hydraulically dissect into the deeper ATCs to communicate with the nasociliary nerve and the oculomotor nerve. It moves superiorly to the superior oblique muscle and the frontal and lacrimal nerves if enough volume is injected. Bulk flow of anesthetic will dissect anteriorly to block the orbicularis fibers as it spreads into both the upper and lower lid if sufficient volume is injected during withdrawal of the needle.

When the medial canthal site is chosen instead of a percutaneous site, there is less chance of bleeding into the lids or deviation of the needle path from squinting. However, a needle no longer than 15 mm should be used if the hub goes deeply enough to touch the conjunctiva of the canthal area. The point should not go beyond the hind surface of the globe or it may enter the medial rectus muscle. Use of a 1″ needle

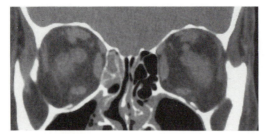

Figure 1.44a.

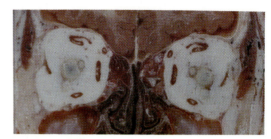

Figure 1.44b.

Figure 1.44. Frontal sections at approximately the hind surface of the eye. Tenon's capsule can be seen in the cryosection and in 1-44c. The ethmoid branch of the ophthalmic artery is about to enter the bone just nasal to the superior oblique muscle. The muscle bellies have not increased much in diameter at this stage, they are still mostly tendinous. The ATCs

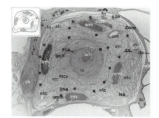

Figure 1.44c.

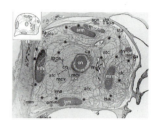

Figure 1.44d.

are very well demarcated and the medial compartment is smaller. Needles should not be placed posterior to this level in the medial compartment because the medial rectus muscle moves toward bone. In the superior nasal compartment the superior ophthalmic vein is beginning to move temporally. There is no intermuscular septum between the lateral rectus muscle and the inferior rectus muscle. The infero-temporal adipose tissue compartment is extensive. Note the subarachnoid space between the optic nerve and the coverings of the nerve.

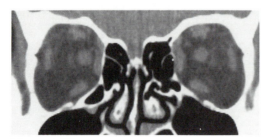

Figure 1.45a.

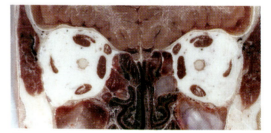

Figure 1.45b.

Figure 1.45. Frontal sections are 3 to 5 mm posterior to the hind surface of the globe. The bellies of the medial, superior, and inferior rectus muscles become much larger. Peribulbarly directed needles could readily enter muscles, which are becoming adherent to the orbital walls. The communicating vein from the facial vein is approaching the superior ophthalmic vein; the latter is moving temporally. The supero-temporal compartment

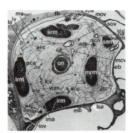

Figure 1.45c.

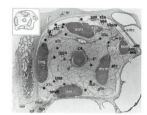

Figure 1.45d.

now starts to fill with blood vessels; the supero-nasal compartment is filled with blood vessels at this level. The central retinal artery can be seen clearly in the center of the optic nerve. Note how well developed the adipose tissue compartments remain. There is no true peribulbar space around the inferior rectus muscle and the lateral rectus muscle.

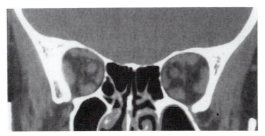

Figure 1.46a.

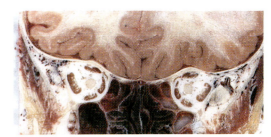

Figure 1.46b.

Figure 1.46c.

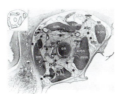

Figure 1.46d.

Figure 1.46. Frontal sections are 9.5 to 12 mm behind the hind surface of the globe. The superior ophthalmic vein is now temporal. The lacrimal artery and vein are in the 10:30 ATC by 8.9 mm behind the hind surface of the eye. Note the branches of the ophthalmic artery in the superior nasal quadrant. The central retinal artery and central retinal vein have left the protection of the optic sheath. The origin of the central retinal artery from the ophthalmic artery occurs in 2 to 3 mm. Thus the area 10 to 12 mm behind the hind surface of the eye is very vulnerable to injury and damage. Septa anchoring the optic nerve to the medial rectus muscle, and to the lateral rectus muscle. The muscles have moved together to make a virtual trap for anesthetics injected in this area. However, injury to the structures is easy. At 12.2 mm behind the hind surface of the eye, notice that the oculomotor nerve branches to the muscles are quite vulnerable to damage by needles, but anesthetics can safely spread into this area.

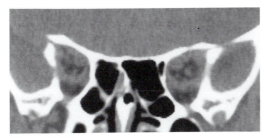

Figure 1.47a.

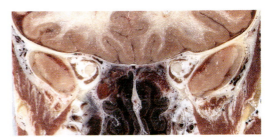

Figure 1.47b.

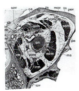

Figure 1.47c.

Figure 1.47d.

Figure 1.47. Frontal sections approaching the orbital apex 15 mm behind the hind surface of the eye to the optic canal at 24.5 mm behind the hind surface of the eye. The muscle cone is fully developed, the muscles are almost contiguous at 15 mm behind the hind surface of the eye—very little space exists for anesthetic to escape. The structures are particularly vulnerable. The ophthalmic artery at 15.5 mm is dividing. All of the motor nerves are approaching the surface of the muscle that they will eventually innervate. Within this 5 mm space, the nerves are vulnerable to anesthetic diffusion. The structures are tightly compressed at 18.4 mm behind the eye, and continue to become more packed as they approach the orbital apex. If the hub of a 35 mm needle is at the equator of an eye of average length whose equator is at the inferior orbital rim, the point of the needle will be 22.5 mm behind the hind surface of the eye.

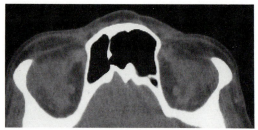

Figure 1.48a.

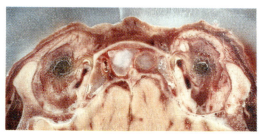

Figure 1.48b.

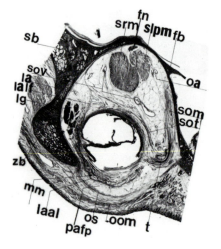

Figure 1.48c.

Figure 1.48. Transverse sections through the upper orbit through the trochlea and superior oblique muscle. Both the tendon and the ophthalmic vein can be easily injured by injections in the supero-nasal compartment. The cryosection shows how large the superior ophthalmic vein is in this quadrant. The ATC supero-temporally appears to be relatively free of structures.

stopping the hub at the intersection of the extended imaginary plane of the iris for an eye of average axial length is recommended.

Injection of local anesthetic in the preseptal space at the medial canthal site will block medial motor fibers to the orbicularis of the upper and lower lid and provide lid and conjunctival anesthesia to the medial aspect of each lid. This injection will anesthetize the canaliculi, puncta, and lacrimal sac.

The superior nasal adipose tissue compartment is relatively unsafe to pass needles through percutaneously because the trochlea crosses it anteriorly, the superior ophthalmic vein goes through it, and the ethmoid and nasal arteries traverse it. However, anesthetics injected there will block the frontal and supratrochlear nerves for conjunctival or lid anesthesia and spread to produce akinesia of the levator, superior rectus, superior oblique, and medial rectus muscles.

Pannu describes filling the orbit from this site and reports total orbital and lid anesthesia and akinesia; however he has returned to the infero-temporal approach. Injection from the supero-nasal site may block the lacrimal nerve, but is not reliable, except with large volume injection. Injection at this site should never block the infraorbital or zygomatic nerves, so complete conjunctival anesthesia should not be expected unless a large volume dissects anteriorly into the preseptal space. Needle damage to the nerves or myotoxic effects to the levator muscle or superior oblique muscle must be considered when using this compartment.

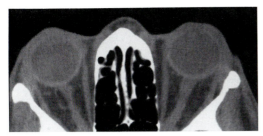

Figure 1.49a.

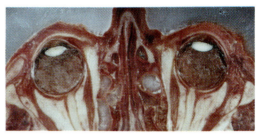

Figure 1.49b.

Figure 1.49. Transverse sections through approximately the center of the lens of the eye and the optic nerve. The optic nerve has been sectioned as it leaves the globe and enters the optic canal. The medial rectus muscle begins to approach bone 5 mm behind the hind surface of the eye, so needles should not be inserted posterior to the hind surface of the eye to provide 5 mm of safety. The expected point of entry into the medial compartment is usually at 3:30 or 4:00 which is somewhat inferior to this actual section and likely inferior to the medial rectus muscle. The lateral rectus muscle is adherent to bone in the mid-orbit .

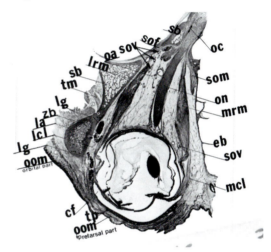

Figure 1.49c.

The infero-nasal compartment can be accessed medially percutaneously at 5:00 or transconjunctivally with 10 degree inferior angulation from the medial canthus as described. The palpebral artery, the angular vein, and the inferior oblique muscle can be injured. Care must be taken to clear the equator of the globe; often the nose is an impediment. When the needle is inferior to the medial rectus muscle and clear of the equator, then it can be angled 10 degrees toward the optical axis and will enter the inferior aspect of the oculomotor compartment for rapid onset of akinesia of the inferior rectus and the inferior oblique muscles.

Compartmentalization of the Mid-Orbit

Figure 1.53 shows the large orbital septal compartments that support and cushion the globe during movement. There is a large compartment intrinsic to each of the rectus muscles as Koornneef's spatial reconstructions demonstrate, and they are interconnected by common septa. Figure 1.54 is a computer reconstruction of the orbits of Figures 1.26 to 1.35 to demonstrate the major and minor septa and the relationship of the septa to the periorbit.

Figure 1.55 is a view of the posterior orbit from behind looking out into the mid-orbit.[17] The septal walls direct the bulk flow of anesthetic, which will readily pass through compartments and between them if the septa are thin or where there are

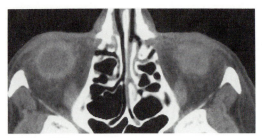

Figure 1.50a.

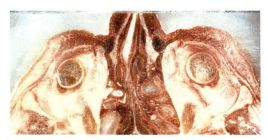

Figure 1.50b.

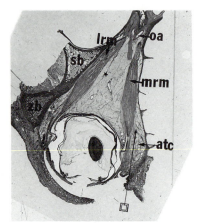

Figure 1.50c.

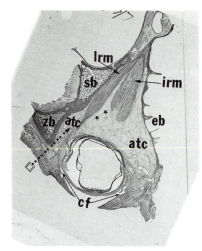

Figure 1.50d.

Figure 1.50. Transverse sections at the inferior limbus. Notice the fatty spaces medial and lateral in the CT and cryosections. The lateral rectus muscle attaches to the bone approximately 5 mm behind the hind surface of the eye, obliterating the periorbital space in that area in the histologic section, which is slightly superior to the cryosection. Medially, there is a fatty space that continues for quite a distance. This is the projected space into which anesthetic will go from the medial compartment .

fenestrations. Septal walls vary in compliance (Figure 1.56); less developed septa with large fenestrations allow the anesthetic solution to be distributed throughout the orbit. Thick septa will compartmentalize the injection, leading to large increases in intraocular pressure even with small injection volumes and to poor distribution of anesthetic about the orbit.[6,17,18] Persons with thick septa are likely to develop blindness as the first symptom of Graves' disease or instead of proptosis.

Artists' drawings suggest that the four rectus muscles are interconnected from their attachments to the globe to the back of the orbit by a common intermuscular septum [43,44] (Figure 1.57) to form a surgical intraconal or retrobulbar space and a peripheral periorbital space. There is no such compartmentalization, as Figure 1.58 shows in contrast.

No such common intermuscular septum exists from approximately 5 mm behind the equator of the eye to the orbital apex except in the supero-temporal quadrant, as serial sectioning of many orbits has shown.[6,12,13]

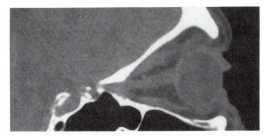

Figure 1.51a.

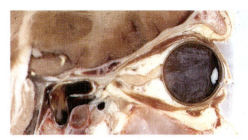

Figure 1.51b.

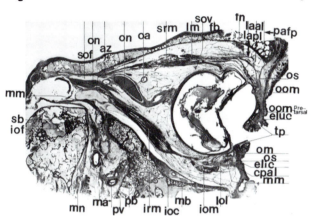

Figure 1.51c.

Figure 1.51. Sagittal sections cut parallel to the optic nerve through the lens and the optic canal. The cryosection, Figure 1.46b, is a very large eye in a very small orbit. The orbital apex of this eye is easily accessible with a 1 1/4″ needle. A needle placed more than 6 or 7 mm from the hind surface of the eye would enter the vascular part of the muscle cone. In the histologic sections, c and d, there is the usual 25 mm retrobulbar space. Note the fatty space above the levator muscle, and the fatty space inferior to the inferior rectus muscle. The orbital septum is much thinner in the inferior lid than in the superior lid, and note the splitting of the upper and lower lid retractors into anterior and posterior lamellae. Imagine the lid retracted for transconjunctival injection; then visualize various transconjunctival needle tracks, as well as the percutaneous tracts.

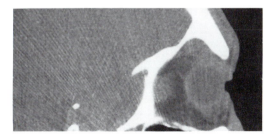

Figure 1.52a.

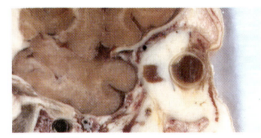

Figure 1.52b.

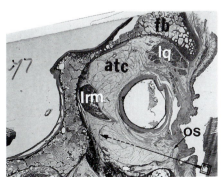

Figure 1.52c.

Figure 1.52. Sagittal sections cut parallel to the optic nerve through the lateral limbus. Observe how much fatty space exists in the infero-temporal compartment and supero-temporally behind the orbital portion of the lacrimal gland. The septa seem to be radial. The orbital septum in the inferior lid is almost non-existent in the histologic section.

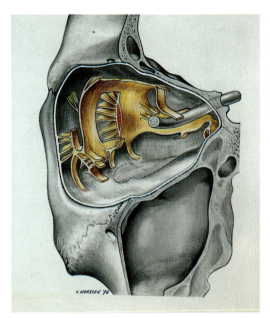

Figure 1.53a. Drawing of the connective tissue of the superior levator palpebrae/superior rectus muscle complex and of the connective tissue of the superior oblique muscle. (With permission from Swets & Zeitlinger BV)

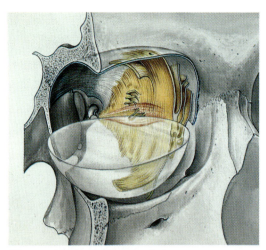

Figure 1.53b. Drawing of the connective tissue system of the medial rectus muscle. (With permission from Swets & Zeitlinger BV)

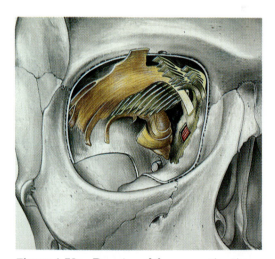

Figure 1.53c. Drawing of the connective tissue of the inferior rectus and inferior oblique muscles. (With permission from Swets & Zeitlinger BV)

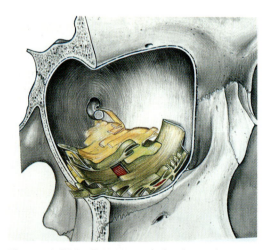

Figure 1.53d. Drawing of the lateral rectus muscle connective tissue apparatus. (With permission from Swets & Zeitlinger BV)

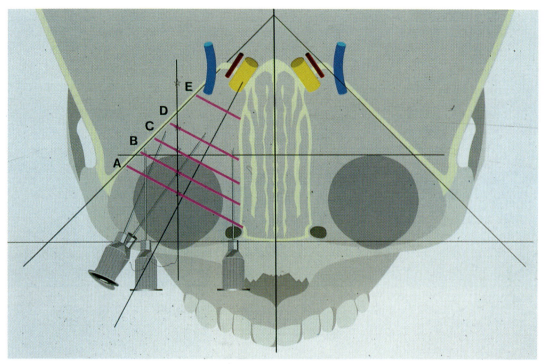

Figure 1.54a.

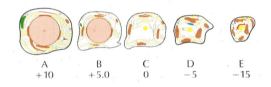

A	B	C	D	E
+10	+5.0	0	−5	−15

Figure 1.54b.

Figure 1.54. Computer-generated reconstruction of the orbital fibrous-muscular apparatus. The large septa have three layers, small septa are single layered. Analysis of these sections should enable the reader to visualize the location of connective tissue, nerves, arteries and veins. These reconstructions will be used in Figure 1.59 to analyze needle paths, flow, and diffusion of local anesthetic agents. (a) Transverse mid-axial plane to show where orbital reconstructions of the septal tissue were performed. (b) Reconstructions of the orbital septal/fibro-muscular tissue; nerves in yellow, arteries in red, and veins in blue.

The septa of the infero-temporal area through which "retrobulbar" needles pass are primarily radial, as they are in the supero-nasal and infero-nasal quadrants. However, minor septa abound forming walls of cellules which offer little impediment to needles, but discourage anesthetic solution from moving freely in the orbit.

The orbit is compartmentalized into an intraconal space only when the closeness of the muscles forms a muscular pocket in the deep or posterior orbit (shown in Figures 1.33 through 1.35). Since the muscles are attached by septa to the periorbit, there is no discrete "periorbital space" or "periconal space," except medial to the medial rectus muscle and supero-temporally peripheral to the septum connecting the superior rectus and the lateral rectus muscle.

Generations of ophthalmologists have believed that when a patient is poorly

Figure 1.55. An artist's depiction of the septa in the posterior orbit viewed from behind looking into the mid-orbit. Note the superior ophthalmic vein coursing from superior-nasal to superior-temporal. Notice the septa between the optic nerve and the medial rectus muscle and the lateral rectus muscle. Note how compartmentalized the orbit leading into the posterior orbit is. Note the "oculomotor compartment," or central compartment, alongside the optic nerve. Injection in this space will touch the branches of the oculomotor nerve, the ciliary nerves, and the ciliary ganglion, whereas the ATCs lateral and medial to it will limit spread of anesthetic, especially in those persons with thick septa. (With permission from MP Bergen, MD and Swets & Zeitlinger, BV—modified)

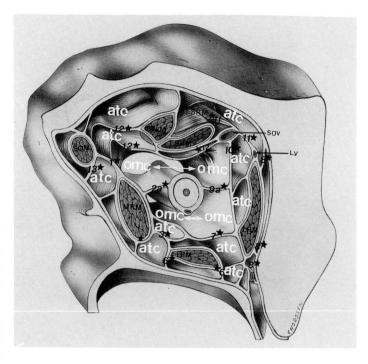

anesthetized or has poor akinesia after a "retrobulbar" block that the injection was not placed into the surgical retrobulbar space due to the failure to penetrate the intermuscular septum between the lateral and inferior rectus muscles. According to such teaching, that septum needed to be penetrated to allow the flow of anesthetics into the retrobulbar space. It has also been taught that blocks which avoided this "retrobulbar space" were "periorbital", "peribulbar" or "periocular".

It is obvious this division of the orbital space does not exist in the infero-temporal area. Therefore, there must be a better anatomical explanation of the variation in block results— not failure to penetrate this septum—and nomenclature of blocks should reflect anatomical facts, such as the site of the needle point at which injection takes place.

Atkinson[23,24] referred to penetrating the orbital septum with one motion of the needle and then directing the patient to look "up and in" to position the needle posterior to the intermuscular septum between the inferior and lateral rectus muscles, to avoid penetrating the intermuscular septum. He recognized that the "intermuscular septum" ceased as the posterior pole of the globe was reached. He referred to his block as cone injection, which would be anatomically correct, unless the needle passed under the optic nerve and out into the space between the medial and superior rectus muscles where it would become "periorbital."

It is easy to place a needle in this medial periorbital space in the fresh cadaver. Injection into this space probably accounts for the failure of some small volume apical or conal anesthetic injections to block the ciliary nerves or the oculomotor nerve.

Why do "experts" in "retrobulbar block" still believe that to have a good block there

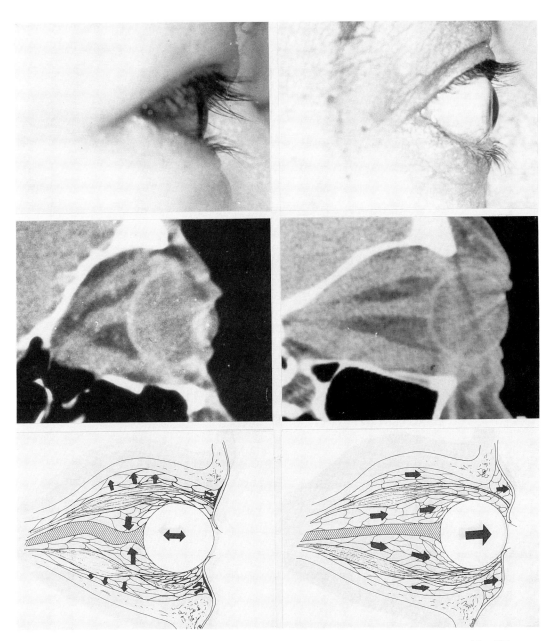

Figure 1.56. Malignant and nonmalignant Graves' Ophthalmology. Patient with profile, CT scans, and schematic drawings. (left Malignant Graves' Ophthalmology. Note the tight connective tissue system preventing the orbital contents and the eye to displace anteriorly, resulting in rise of intraorbital pressure. Right) Nonmalignant, proptotic Graves' Ophthalmology. (With permission from Blackwell Scientific Publications)

Figure 1.57. Frontal section of right orbit posterior to the globe demonstrating intermuscular septum, which ensheathes the rectus muscles. (With permission from Jeffrey Koziol, MD and WB Saunders Co.)

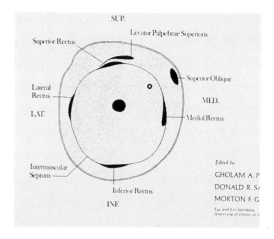

Figure 1.58. Histologic section shows no intermuscular septum ensheathing the rectus muscle and connecting them to each other posterior to the hind surface of the globe.

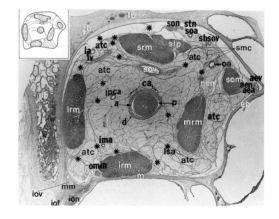

should be a "pop" as the needle goes through the intermuscular septum into the magic space?

The minor septa which divide the inferotemporal adipose compartment into many antero-posterior subdivisions are no impediment to even a fairly dull needle and do not "pop." However, injection in the more peripheral cells encourages the solution to stay more lateral in the septal compartment next to the "periorbit" as seen in Figure 1.55, rather than encouraging spread more centrally down into the central or oculomotor compartment—resulting in poor or slow blocks of the oculomotor nerve.

Septa adjacent to the sclera "pop," as do robust areas of the capsulopalpebral fascia, which attach Tenon's to the periorbit: these should "pop." These structures should keep the needle close to the globe and direct anesthetic solution into the central adipose compartment alongside the globe and optic nerve.

There are sizeable septa adjacent to the globe in the mid-orbit, which a needle would "pop" between the inferior oblique muscle and the inferior rectus muscle, between the inferior oblique muscle and the lateral rectus muscle, between the inferior rectus muscle and the medial rectus muscle, and between the medial rectus muscle and Muller's muscle. These septa are very close to the globe (shown in Figures 1.28 and 1.29). A needle trajectory close to the globe, aimed at the orbital apex, puts anesthetic in the central compartment alongside the optic nerve. Needle tracks close to the globe, which encourage the straight needle to continue on close to the optic nerve provide a more direct path to the oculomotor nerve area, but put the optic nerve at risk.

Septa also exist deeper in the orbit between the medial rectus muscle and the optic nerve; between the inferior rectus muscle and the optic nerve; and between the lateral rectus muscle and the optic nerve (shown in Figures 1.30 through 1.32). Additionally, septa support veins that run between the optic nerve and both the lateral and inferior rectus muscles. Penetration of these septa should cause a "pop." Finally, there is a septum posteriorly between the inferior rectus muscle and Muller's muscle. Anesthetic injected in this region should be close to the oculomotor nerve and the ciliary ganglion. Rapid anesthesia and akinesia should occur, but so can injury to arteries, veins, nerves, and the optic sheath if the orbit is shallow.

Since any "pop" could signify an injury to a vulnerable structure, a different approach is suggested. Follow the ATCs without creating a "pop", stop in the mid-orbit and let the fluid do the dissection. Swan[45] and O'Brien[46] suggest terminology and logic for placing needles in the anterior mid-orbit allowing the fluid to dissect. This approach makes good anatomic sense.

Anesthetics injected in the mid-orbit bathe the ciliary nerves, which traverse the mid-orbit.[45] Injectate may spread into the muscular cone to bathe the motor nerve fasciculi and the ciliary ganglion of a shallow orbit, or it may spread primarily peripherally or anteriorly in a deep orbit producing minimal ocular akinesia. However, the efferent fibers of the ciliary ganglion and the sensory fibers to the globe will be blocked in the mid-orbit of large or small orbits because the fibers are so small and void of connective tissue covering over a 10 mm length for excellent contact with anesthetic. Inadequate contact of anesthetic with branches of the oculomotor nerve in deep orbits can be readily diagnosed and anesthetic placed deeper in the ATC or in an adjacent ATC to promote total akinesia.

Attempting akinesia from two mid-orbital injection sites has two advantages over seeking it deep in the posterior orbit with a single small volume injection.

Small volume injection in the posterior orbit to block the oculomotor nerve means that the needle must be deep in the posterior orbit very close to the optic nerve, ophthalmic artery, and ophthalmic vein where damage is more likely.[47] It may block the oculomotor nerve, and may miss many sensory fibers. Mid-orbital injection from two sites will augment both the oculomotor block and block the sensory fibers in the respective areas.[48a,48b,49]

The depth of the mid-orbit and the pathway of the septa determine where the anesthetic will go unless needles deep in the muscular cone almost touch the oculomotor nerve. There are shallow and deep orbits. The mid-orbit is subject to considerable volume and septal variation, and the septa vary in robustness and fenestrations. These are the major factors in the variability of akinesia, not failure to penetrate the intermuscular septum between the inferior rectus and lateral rectus muscles in the mid-orbit—a septum which does not anatomically exist.

An incomplete block from a safe, well placed injection is no calamity; it tells the discerning blocker much about the orbit and where to add additional volume.

The Posterior Orbit

The posterior orbit begins where the space between the extraocular muscles is less than one-half the breadth of the muscle, or at about 10 mm from the hind surface of the globe (as seen in Figures 1.33 through 1.35). It ends at the optic canal where the dura splits—the parietal layer to fuse with periosteum to become the "periorbit" and the visceral layer to cover the optic nerve and to continue forward as Tenon's capsule. The muscles, blood vessels, nerves, and connective tissue thus lie in an interdural space analogous to the epidural space of the vertebral column. The two layers of the dura fuse at the apex of the orbit in the same way fusion occurs at the foramen magnum. The epidural space of the orbit thus contains muscles and connective tissue as well as fat and blood vessels. The anterior boundary of the orbital epidural space is the orbital septum/capsulopalpebral fascia complex.

Zinn's annulus attaches to the periorbit at the apex; the extraocular muscles attach to it and to periorbit. The apex is filled with muscles, blood vessels and nerves (seen in Figure 1.24).

A pocket, the muscular cone, exists in the posterior orbit into which anesthetics can be injected into a definite intraconal space. The muscles forming the cone have dense fascial attachments to the periorbit in the posterior orbit so no discrete periorbital space exists between muscles and the periorbit except in two areas: (1) medial to the medial rectus muscle (shown in Figures 1.28 through 1.31 and Figures 1.43 and 1.44) where an ATC is the posterior continuation of the medial ATC along which anesthetics can travel toward the oculomotor and trochlear nerves from injection in the mid-orbit medial ATC (see Figures 1.28 through 1.33); and (2) superior and temporal to the superior rectus (shown in Figure 1.32 through 1.35). This space is closed from the cone by the dense facial attachments between the superior rectus and lateral rectus muscles in the posterior orbit.

Importantly, anesthetics injected in the cone can exit anteriorly and posteriorly between the medial rectus and the superior rectus to reach the medial compartment. This deep supero-nasal ATC is an important exit from the cone because veins in it communicate anteriorly with the facial veins to allow diffusion of fluids if the orbital veins are collapsed in the apex. If this exit was blocked by thick septa or scar tissue an almost closed compartment of small volume would form.

Through the deep supero-nasal ATC anesthetics can travel between the cone and the medial ATC in contact with the oculomotor and nasociliary nerve, and travel toward the frontal, lacrimal, and trochlear nerves (as seen in Figure 1.36).

Anesthetic injected in the infero-temporal compartment in deep orbits may never penetrate deeply enough into the cone to access the oculomotor nerve unless a volume adequate for that patient has been chosen. Thus arose the dangerous incentive to put longer needles more deeply into the cone and to routinely inject large volumes in the deep cone to cover all the nerves.

Note in Figure 1.24 how congested the superonasal quadrant of the posterior orbit is with many arteries; the histologic sections do not give an adequate impression. Damage to any of the arteries in this space could lead to "retrobulbar hemorrhage." This alone should be incentive to avoid injections deep in the orbit in this quadrant. The optic nerve is readily accessible in this quadrant also.

Note that structures in the muscular cone are tightly packed with minimal adipose tissue to absorb local anesthetic or cushion needles. At risk are muscles, veins, arteries, and nerves which can be traumatized when needles intrude. If the septal tissues are non-compliant the veins can be compressed leading to an increase in retinal vein pressure; higher pressure can occlude arteries. High pressure causes a gradient for flow of anesthetic into the optic nerve sheath, if the smallest hole has been sustained in the dura. This can lead to subdural or subarachnoid spread of local anesthetic into the chiasm.

The central retinal vein is vulnerable where it exits the dural sheath to drain posteriorly (as shown in Figure 1.32). The ophthalmic artery is very vulnerable just before its central retinal branch enters the optic nerve and as the artery crosses over the optic nerve because of fascial attachments of the artery to the optic nerve sheath and the annulus (as seen in Figures 1.32 and 1.54 d,e).

The superior orbital vein is exceptionally vulnerable in the temporal aspect after it passes from the mid-orbit (as shown in Figures 1.3 and 1.32) into the posterior orbit (which can be seen in Figures 1.33 and 1.54 d,e). Note the many communicating branches in Figure 1.33. Therefore, supero-temporal injections should not be placed deeper than 5 mm behind the hind surface of the eye to protect this vein. Measure with reference to the globe, not the superior orbital ridge. The needle in the supero-temporal quadrant should never go into the posterior orbit; in a shallow orbit it may be in the cavernous sinus.

The optic nerve is vulnerable in the posterior orbit and the subarachnoid space can be entered through the optic sheath (seen in Figure 1.30 through 1.33). The optic nerve sheath is tethered in the posterior orbit where it is easily entered and the optic nerve penetrated and damaged.[47]

The optic sheath can also be entered in the mid-orbit. It has been entered 5 mm behind the eye using curved needle technique.[50] Drysdale entered it 8 mm behind the eye in his classic paper,[51] and it has been entered with a 25 mm straight needle during peribulbar block in a confidential report to one of the authors. Injection of anesthetic into the sheath can produce subdural or subarachnoid spread of anesthetic. Short beveled needles are more likely to allow the entire injection to go into either space; longer beveled needles are more likely to allow perforation and most of the anesthetic to exit the bevel into the surrounding area. A hole in the sheath followed by injection outside the sheath can lead to a slower onset of brainstem anesthesia.

The branches of the oculomotor nerve are accessible in the posterior orbit for a distance of 5 to 10 mm for contact with anesthetic solutions. The lateral branch of the inferior division to the inferior oblique muscle has an additional 25 mm exposure as it passes forward through the central adipose area to reach the inferior oblique muscle.[52]

Branches of the oculomotor nerve and the muscular artery to each muscle can be readily injured in the hilum area of each muscle where the nerve and artery enter (as seen in Figures 1.32 and 1.33). The muscles are all closely adherent to bone by tight septa in the area of their respective hilum; the hilum for all, except the inferior oblique, is in the posterior orbit. The inferior rectus, medial rectus, superior rectus muscle, and the levator can be left paretic after "retrobulbar block" by this mechanism. The hilum of the inferior oblique can be injured with peribulbar or retrobulbar technique when the track of the needle is in line with the lateral limbus and close to the floor of the orbit. It is tethered as it approaches the muscle in the anterior orbit, so that it is more easily injured. A needle route lateral would seem indicated.

The trochlear nerve and the hilum of the superior oblique are vulnerable at 1:00 to 2:00 in the "periorbital space"—care is indicated in this locus because the muscle is fixed in the supero-temporal orbit. The trochlear nerve can be accessed by anesthetic placed in the medial ATC.

The nasociliary nerve enters the orbit lateral to the ophthalmic artery (as seen in Figures 1.34 and 1.54), rapidly goes medial toward it (shown in Figures 1.35 and 1.54) where it sends branches to the ciliary ganglion, and continues medially where it gives off long ciliary branches and then enters the mid-orbit. The ciliary ganglion and its fibers are vulnerable in the posterior orbit. There are reports of permanent damage to the ciliary ganglion from retrobulbar block.

The ethmoid, infratrochlear, and nasal branches of the nasociliary nerve are readily blocked in the medial compartment in the mid-orbit, so there is no indication to place a needle deep in the posterior orbit to block these nerves.

At this point it is wise to review the structures which do not pass through the cone of muscles—namely, the frontal nerve, the lacrimal nerve, the infraorbital nerve, and the zygomatic nerve. All of these sensory nerves carry branches to the conjunctiva and the lids. One should not expect to block these sensory nerves in the posterior orbit with small injections of "retrobulbar" anesthetic solution, although they should be blocked by medial and lateral orbital blocks. They are easily blocked in the anterior orbit with periocular or peribulbar technique. Blocking these nerves by continuous bathing of the conjunctiva with topical anesthetic can produce only short duration, superficial anesthesia and subjects the corneal epithelium to chemical injury.

Anatomic/Anesthetic Considerations in the Orbit

The flow of an anesthetic solution after it leaves the tip of a needle is very complex (Figure 1.59a-i). In Figure 1.59a, the orbit is imaged in mid-transverse section and the sites are depicted for the Koornneef frontal sections cut perpendicular to the optic nerve. Frontal sections were placed in the skull, a globe suspended in front, then needles were passed to contact the sections to verify measurements and to simulate clinical technique.

The silhouette of needles on Figure 1.59a is based on camera reproductions of the needles with respect to the inferior orbital rim for Atkinson and Gills/Loyd techniques, the plane of the iris for Hustead technique, and the skin for periocular or peribulbar blocks. The sections A, B, C, D, and E are computer reconstructions of the orbital fibromuscular (septa) tissues, arteries, veins, and nerves seen at that section.

In Figures 1.59a-i, the path of needles and bulk flow of anesthetic for a number of anesthetic techniques is traced. Needles start above or below the limbus, whereas the silhouettes are projected to the mid-transverse plane. The needle point moves toward the mid-axis as the needle is moved progressively into the orbit for techniques in which the needle changes planes. The mid-axial plane silhouette is corrected for change of distance as a function of angle of inclination to the transverse plane, but that is only 2 mm in 25 mm at 30°.

In Figure 1.59b-i, a retrobulbar needle is placed according to the technique of Atkinson, a needle at the 8:00 position using the approximate angulation of Hustead, a medial compartment needle intersecting the plane of the iris, a supero-temporal needle

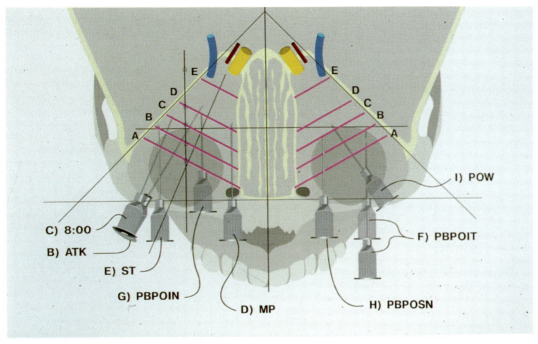

Figure 1.59a (top)

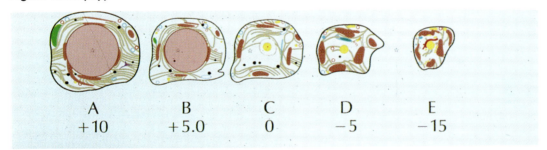

Figure 1.59a (bottom)

Figure 1.59a. Transverse mid-axial computer-generated views of the orbit with the inferior and superior orbital rims silhouetted. Needles were placed in loci according to the published techniques of various authors and photographed from above. The trajectory of the needles in the mid-axial plane were generated. Thus, a 35-mm needle midway between the inferior and lateral rectus muscles at the inferior orbital rim directed superiorly and medially with its path toward the orbital apex is the silhouette in Figure 1.59a labelled "ATK," whose needle points are then transferred into Figure 1.59b to show where the Atkinson needle would travel going through the frontal sections. In each site an injection of 4 ml of anesthetic is held constant and the path and change in concentration of the anesthetic depicted with the following assumptions: (1) that anesthetic will pass through minor septa (single line of septal tissue) with minimal delay, but that major septa (depicted as three lines of septal connective tissue) will cause diversion and redistribution of anesthetic; (2) that the force of injection through a small needle will take the anesthetic preferentially in the posterior direction until sufficient resistance is met to cause it to come anteriorly; (3) the concentration will decreqse by 50% for each 10 mm of posterior movement and for each 5 mm of anterior movement; and (4) that once an orbital decompression device is applied the fluids will distribute throughout the minor septal compartments, thus going more central or laterally or anteriorly, but will hesitate to cross major septa, although diffusion will proceed at a much slower rate.

Figure 1.59b. A computer simulation of anesthetic flow labeled "ATK."

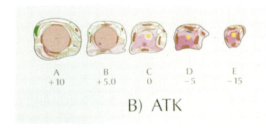

Figure 1.59c. 31.7 mm needle inserted at 8:00 travelling 30° medially to the sagittal plane to make an angle of 30° with the optical axis and directed 5-10° superiorly is labelled "8:00," to duplicate where Hustead places needles in the infero-temporal quadrant.

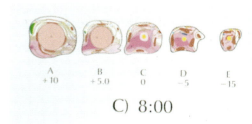

Figure 1.59d. "Medial pericone needle" placed in the medial compartment through the medial canthal angle.

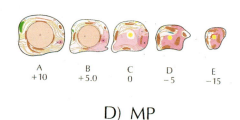

Figure 1.59e. 25 mm needle in the supero-temporal technique of Thornton.

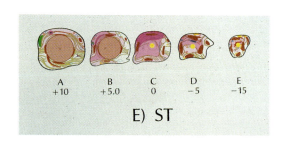

Figure 1.59f. 21 mm needle placed infero-temporally described in peribulbar blocks by Davis '90 or Wang (Wang uses 25 mm of a 38 mm needle to end 1 to 2 mm posterior to the hind surface of the eye).

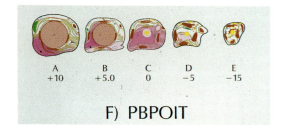

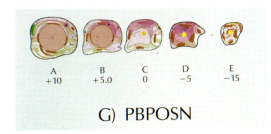

Figure 1.59g. Supero-nasal injection site of Davis using a 7/8″ needle pushed until the hub touches the upper lid crease.

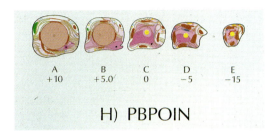

Figure 1.59h. Infero-nasal periocular block position pushing a 7/8″ needle until the skin of the inferior lid crease is taught.

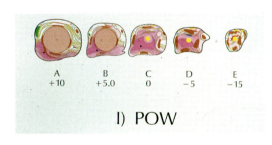

Figure 1.59i. Position of Weiss infero-temporally pushing a 7/8″ needle to its hub until the skin overlying the globe is tense.

with the hub intersecting the plane of the iris. Peribulbar injections according to Davis '90 and periocular needles according to Bloomberg and Weiss are shown. For demonstration, the shorter needle was inserted to the equator because the skin allows the hub to travel well past the equator in more than 75% of patients.

Note in the cross-sections A, B, C, D, and E the approximate end points of the needle tip if its hub is at a given locus, then follow bulk flow of anesthetic from the needles in their respective sections.

In the diagrams, it is assumed that for persons with ordinary septal size, fluid would flow through the minor septa (single line in graphics) with minor delay or loss of concentration. However, major redistribution would take place at major septa (3 septal lines in the graphics). As the solution moves through the adipose compartments, much loss of concentration would occur by dilution and absorption. Dilution to 50% was assumed as the 5 ml volume traveled 10 mm in the direction of flow or 5 mm backwards. Radioisotope labelling will be necessary to establish a better approximation.

Note the subtle similarities and the minor differences with the different anesthetic techniques.

Koornneef predicted in 1974 that anesthetics would spread throughout the orbit in many orbits when injected in adequate volume in the anterior orbit, the mid-orbit, or in the posterior orbit, and that the final effect after the spread phase would be indistinguishable by frontal x-ray examination. This has been confirmed in CT scans by Sappo and Nikki[53] for periocular and retrobulbar blocks by Vogl.[54] The (Figure 1.60) radio-opaque tracer moves into all the "retrobulbar" and "periorbital" spaces. Small volume injection in the muscle cone remained localized in the compartment of injection.(Figure 1.61)[54]

Pressure is a function of the compliance of the system, the force available for injection, the volume injected, and the rate of injection. When fluid volume is injected into any orbital compartment a pressure gradient ensues. When a pressure gradient exists, the fluid flows along septa. Some dissolves in the tissues and some passes through fenestrations into other compartments. When the pressure of the bolus reaches the pressure of the tissue, fluid stops moving through the tissues. Fluid pressure will then gradually return to baseline as shown by Otto.[55]

The potential force available is the energy of the thumb depressing the plunger of the syringe—less than or equal to 200 mm Hg with a 5 ml syringe or 1000 mm Hg with a 1-ml syringe. Force exerted in the tissues depends upon the volume injected, the rate of injection, and the distensibility of the tissues. The latter will depend upon the volume of the orbit and the distensibility of the septa.

If the volume of the orbit is great enough in a compliant orbit and the rate of injection is slow enough, there will be minimal pressure rise.

The anesthetic will flow posteriorly, superiorly, inferiorly, laterally, medially, and finally anteriorly where it will flow through fenestrations in the orbital septum to anesthetize the small nerves of the overlying orbicularis muscle. Duke-Elder[56] believes a pressure of 40 to 50 mm Hg is necessary for fluid dissection from the mid-orbit through the orbital septum. The actual reference by Heerfordt[57] showed a range of 10-120 with air as the dissecting medium in cadavers; high pressure was necessary in younger individuals; dissection occurred at the much lower pressure of 10 mm Hg in older patients. Fluid dissection with saline solution should occur at a lower pressure than air because no air/fluid interface is formed; blood requires higher pressure because it does not readily flow through tissue interfaces and is more viscous. No data on this subject in the orbit have been published to our knowledge.

Tight orbits or those orbits with tight septal compartments with compact, nonfenestrated septa can be readily pressurized to 100 mm Hg with anesthetic injection, because of the force exerted on the plunger of the syringe. Such force will collapse the orbital veins and can exceed central retinal artery pressure if the fluid cannot be absorbed or escape into other compartments. Salt solutions are readily absorbed if the veins are open, but absorption should stop if the veins are compressed. These tight orbits are at risk from blindness with Graves' disease, retrobulbar hemorrhage, trauma, or blepharoplasty.[14,58] Persons with small, tight orbits must be made aware of this possibility.

Information about tight orbits is available to those injecting anesthetic if they feel the globe with the free hand, while injecting anesthetic. The feel of "compliance pressure" from anesthetic injected in the posterior orbit with tight septa can be learned; it is not equal to the force exerted on the plunger of the syringe.

Injection into tight orbits markedly increases intraocular pressure as it compresses veins before being sensed as resistance to injection through the syringe. Orbits have been observed in which the globe became firm with 2.5 ml of fluid injected in the mid-orbit. Such orbits, if subject to more volume, stay at a pressure exceeding retinal perfusion

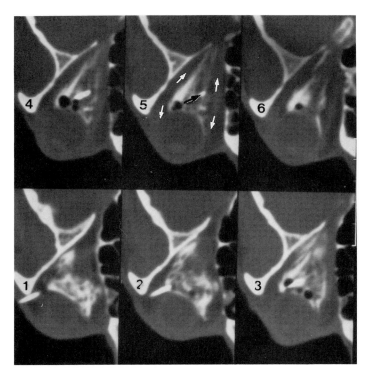

Figure 1.60a. Transverse CT scan with contrast medium fills the intra- and extraconal spaces two minutes after the retrobulbar injection of 3 ml solution. #1 is inferior at the level of the inferior limbus and #6 above the superior limbus. The origin and insertion of the lateral and medial rectus muscles are indicated by small white arrows. (Courtesy G. Vogl, MD)

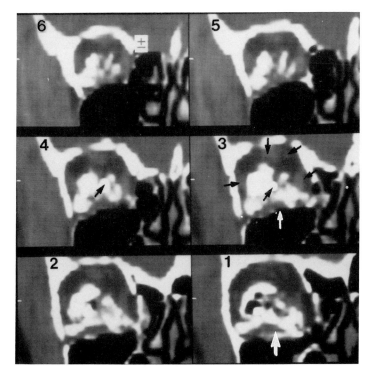

Figure 1.60b. Coronal reconstruction of the above #1 is at the hind surface of the globe and #1 is at the hind surface of the globe and #6 20 mm posterior. The insertion of the inferior oblique is the large white arrow in b-1; the inferior rectus is the small white arrow; the remaining EOMs are labelled with black arrows. (Courtesy G. Vogl, MD)

Figure 1.60c. Sagittal reconstruction parallel to the optic nerve. View 1 is most lateral, proceeding medially at 2.2 mm until 6, which is just medial to the insertion of the medial rectus muscle (Courtesy G. Vogl, MD).

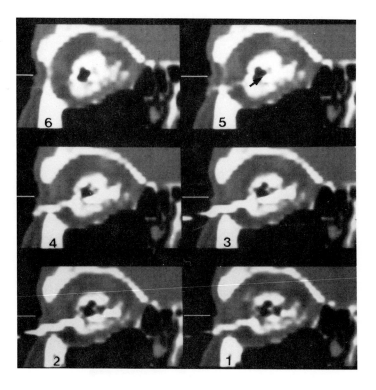

pressure if the globe is not subject to intermittent digital massage because the veins are compressed and there are no lymphatics in the mid- or posterior orbit to remove fluid.[59]

Orbital massage could be vision-saving if it allows even a small amount of fluid to move across septa into areas where the veins are open when the digital pressure is reduced, or through fenestrations in the orbital septum out into the veins and lymphatics of the anterior orbit. Canthotomy and septotomy would be mandatory if blood instead of fluid was the problem because blood cannot be reabsorbed into the veins. The use of the smallest possible needle, avoiding needle placement in the posterior orbit, staying clear of the arteries and veins of the mid-orbit, and injecting slowly while feeling globe pressure should minimize injury.

Anesthetic diffuses into tissues during the bulk spread phase, which decreases the concentration of agent as it moves in the orbit. In proportion there is much more tissue to take up anesthetic than there is nerve to absorb it—the non-nervous tissue has a high affinity for anesthetic solution. Furthermore, the orbit has very rapid blood flow which removes anesthetic even during bulk flow. These two factors make orbital regional anesthesia qualitatively different from any other regional anesthetic procedure. Even though the anesthetic is injected in the epidural space of the orbit, there are significant differences between orbital and vertebral epidural anesthesia.

After bulk flow ceases in the orbital epidural space, diffusion of remaining drug will continue until equilibrium is established or vascular absorption is complete.

Akinesia of the various extraocular muscles may be qualitatively different from a single injection in one part of the orbit since anesthetic is absorbed during movement of the bulk phase. These phenomena as well as septal distributions will influence the

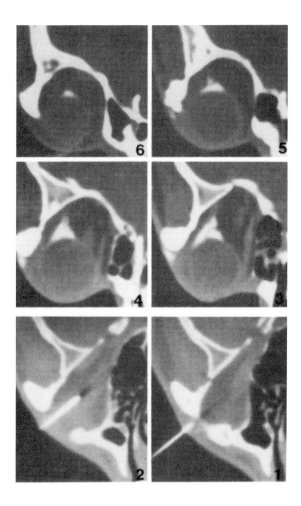

Figure 1.61. Small volume injection in the center of the muscle cone. Note how compartmentalized the injection remains. (Courtesy of G. Vogl, MD)

concentration of drug in the abducens, trochlear, or various branches of the oculomotor nerves.

There is great variability in achieving akinesia with retrobulbar or peribulbar single injection technique. Failure to produce akinesia means that anesthetic has not diffused into the oculomotor nerve or its fasciculi in high enough concentration to block a sufficient length of the nerve or to penetrate to the center of it (see Chapter 2). It is not uncommon to have no akinesia from a 4 or 5 ml injection in some patients or total akinesia after an injection of 1.5 ml to 2 ml. Most likely the former injection entered the mid-orbit, while the latter entered deeply into an oculomotor compartment (Figure 1.55).

The effect of a given volume of anesthetic solution in producing akinesia is a direct measurement of the proximity of the injection to the oculomotor compartment, to the "tightness" of the cone in retaining it to increase diffusion toward the oculomotor nerves, and, inversely, to the volume of the mid-orbit.

Anesthetic given in the mid-orbit spreads and diffuses in all directions and may or may not move posteriorly enough in high enough concentration to block the myelinated oculomotor nerve which is covered by a thick perineurium over the 5 to 7 mm length of exposure. To get total akinesia, 5 to 7 nodes of Ranvier must be blocked in myelinated nerves, which is 3 to 7 mm in length.[10] A small volume (1 ml) injection close enough to the division of the oculomotor nerve should block all branches as Gifford showed by hydraulic dissection with rounded point needles placed deep into the apex.[33] There is no justification to put needles so deeply in the orbit; if they are placed that deeply they should be dulled in the maneuver Gifford discussed and fluid should be injected ahead of the needle after it is 5 to 8mm behind the hind surface of the globe.

We believe that there is an oculomotor compartment in the sense that anesthetics can track along the septa back to the origins of the oculomotor nerve; this is inferred from anesthetic injection and analysis of the orbital reconstructions (shown in Figures 1.37, 1.38, and 1.55). Needle entrance into this compartment will produce rapid akinesia and transmit considerable anesthetic solution into the branches. Unfortunately for patient safety, the oculomotor compartment is very close to the optic nerve.

Further reconstructions will be necessary to study the connective tissue and septa of the oculomotor nerve branches in enough detail to outline a specific oculomotor compartment and to see its relationship with the abducens and ciliary nerves. This is an area ripe for future study.

The oculomotor compartment is accessible without perforating major septa infero-temporally, infero-nasally, and supero-nasally in the mid-orbit, but, supero-temporally in the mid-orbit only after penetrating the septum between the lateral rectus muscle and the superior rectus/levator complex.

The superior oblique muscle and the trochlear nerve are in their own compartment which can be entered by diffusion in the mid-orbit by anesthetic percutaneously supero-temporally or supero-nasally, medially, or through the deep posterior superonasal compartment. The added risk of the supero-nasal route has been discussed.

Incomplete akinesia in any muscular compartment can be converted to complete akinesia by supplemental injection of anesthetic solution in the adipose tissue compartment adjacent to the muscle or septal compartment which was not blocked. Incomplete akinesia may be overcome by augmentation, that is, by repeating the injection while there is still anesthetic in the tissues surrounding the nerves. This latter method is not always as satisfactory as the first. Occasionally, both methods will be necessary to produce absolute akinesia.

If injections in the orbit are made only with reference from the bony contours of the orbit—for example, always from the inferior orbital rim at the intersection of the medial 2/3 and lateral 1/3—and a certain length needle is always inserted until the hub touches the orbital rim, no relationship can be made between volume used and the distance of the needle from the cone or orbital apex since the globe may be very anterior in some people and very posterior in others, as shown in Figures 1.7 and 1.8.

If, however, the length of the needle is known and the length of the globe is known, then the position of the needle in the orbit can be inferred within several millimeters (as seen in Figure 1.59). A given volume of anesthetic injected into the same locus in all persons will, therefore, give some evidence as to the length or volume of the orbit and/or the "tightness of the cone." The chosen site of injection should be shallow enough not to enter the apex of shallow orbits which can be easily injured with average length needles inserted from bony landmarks. One author spots the needle point 5 to 8 mm behind the hind surface of the eye at the intersection of the extended sagittal plane of the lateral limbus.

The authors believe that any time 3.5 ml cannot be injected over 30 seconds without pressure build-up in the globe, the patient has a tight cone or a shallow orbit, or both. This occurs in about 5% of orbits. Rapid akinesia is the rule in such orbits from this volume of anesthetic, as if minimal tissue existed to absorb anesthetic except for the oculomotor nerve. As yet radiographic or MRI substantiation of orbital size or distance to the cone in these individuals is not available.

One author finds that 50% of globes will be totally akinetic and some 40% of orbits will require an additional injection in an adjacent compartment to complete total akinesia. This is achieved with minimal pressure rise with 3.5 ml of a mixture of 2% mepivacaine/0.75% bupivacaine injected in the infero-temporal compartment with the needle point placed 5 to 8 mm behind the hind surface of the eye. In 5% of orbits the injection was stopped at 3.0 ml because of pressure rising.

Some 5% of patients will require injection in three quadrants and/or additional infero-temporal injection 5 to 10 mm deeper in order to obtain complete akinesia. Obviously, these latter patients have very large orbits, very "loose" cones, very rapid uptake of anesthetic, or septa which prevent entrance of anesthetic into the oculomotor compartment. Such information is useful in the block of the fellow eye.

Sensory nerves to the globe, the ciliary nerves, pass through the mid-orbit and are readily blocked by anesthetics injected in the space behind the globe or along side the globe, or in the sub-Tenon's, or subcapsular spaces. However, conjunctival sensory fibers are missed by such injection, as is well known, since the ciliary nerves innervate the cornea and only 3 to 4 mm from the limbus.

Sensory fibers to the conjunctiva stem from the nasociliary nerve, which may be incompletely blocked in the mid-orbit, and the frontal nerve, the lacrimal nerve, the infra-orbital nerve, and the zygomatic nerve, which do not pass through the mid-orbit in the space behind the eye or in the sub-Tenon's space, as they are anatomically separated from the cone in the deep orbit (as shown in Figure 1.35).

Thus anesthesia of the globe does not imply anesthesia of the conjunctiva, nor does akinesia of the globe. Small volume injections in the mid-orbit may produce spotty or no subconjunctival anesthesia, as well as incomplete akinesia.

Anesthetic must be placed in the proper locus to block the sensory nerves of the conjunctiva. This is accomplished by superficial injection of anesthetic in the quadrants of the anterior orbit or by blocking the sensory nerves deep in the mid orbit—inside the cone or in the medial compartment for the nasociliary and outside the muscle cone for the lacrimal and frontal, and outside the orbit for branches of the infraorbital and zygomatic or inside the infraorbital canal.

The supero-temporal route usually will block the frontal and lacrimal nerves and, if the septum is penetrated by the needle, the injection will block all the nasociliary as well as the motor nerves of the orbit as noted by Thornton in Chapter 3 and Kelman.[39]

The branches of the infraorbital and zygomatic nerves are easily and safely blocked after they emerge from their respective foramina. Anesthetic of sufficient concentration injected into the lower lid in the preseptal space will usually diffuse to block them, as in a Van Lint block, or by bulk spread from periocular, peribulbar, or Gills/Loyd blocks. Thus akinesia of the lower lid is usually associated with anesthesia of the conjunctiva and lid, except medially where the infratrochlear nerve makes considerable contribution. The infratrochlear branch is accessible in the supero-nasal compartment or the medial compartment of the anterior orbit as it emerges to innervate the conjunctiva and lids.

Akinesia of the upper lid is rarely associated with conjunctival anesthesia or sensory anesthesia of the upper lid when obtained by a Van Lint block of the upper lid. This is because most of the sensory supply is from branches of the frontal and infratrochlear nerves which innervate the lid more medially. The Van Lint block reaches only the lacrimal and zygomatic contributions to the lid.

The parasympathetic nerves to the orbit pass through the ciliary ganglion which is approximately 15 mm from the hind surface of the eye; the ganglion and fibers leaving or passing through it are easily anesthetized by injections in the mid-orbit.

Sympathetic nerves to the orbit do not follow the carotid or ophthalmic arteries.[60] They join the branches of the third, fourth, fifth, sixth, and seventh nerves and distribute along to the muscles and to segments of the eye and lids.[60] Thus, when total akinesia of the eye and lids exists, a total sympathetic block can be expected. Without total akinesia, the sympathetics may not be totally blocked and the patient may develop visceral pain, nausea, cardiovascular problems, or orbital congestion.

Complete akinesia of the globe is believed to lessen the likelihood of choroidal effusion because it prevents muscle pull on the sclera.[33,61] This may be due to the completeness of the sympathetic block, as much or more than the block of the extraocular muscles. Because the sympathetic nerves are in the periphery of the extraocular muscles, and do not have the same heavy myelin sheath as do motor fibers, they may be fully blocked when the more central motor nerves are only partially blocked. This matter of sympathetic block of the orbit is worthy of further pharmacologic and anatomic study.

It is possible to have total akinesia of the eye from "retrobulbar anesthesia" in a patient who still feels pain from cataract surgery unless the conjunctiva is bathed by topical anesthetic or blocked by subconjunctival injection of local anesthetics, as recommended by Atkinson.[23,24] The patient with a mid-orbital block or "periorbital" or "periocular" block may feel no pain when the conjunctiva is excised or the iris manipulated, and yet the globe will be moving.

Patient acceptance of peribulbar and periocular blocks is high due to lack of pain with surgery, but the moving globe may cause the surgeon anxiety.

It is possible to please both the patient and surgeon by injecting suitable supplemental injections delivered to the correct anatomic site in adequate volume. Such supplemental injections can be made before surgery for a more comfortable patient, better autonomic control, and postoperative analgesia.

It is very important to understand the relationship of needle paths to the production of pain. Certain structures in the orbit can be touched with no sensation by the patient, other structures produce severe pain.

Facial skin and conjunctiva have a high concentration of sensory nerves—injections there are usually considered quite painful. The most painful part of most block techniques occurs when anesthetic is injected into the conjunctiva or into the skin of the eyelids or face to produce lid akinesia or anesthesia. It is possible to prevent this pain by very slow injection or by diluting anesthetics with BSS[62a,b] so that pain receptors are not activated during injection; the combination will produce painless anesthesia and akinesia of the lid.

Periosteum and sclera have a high number of pain receptors. Touching or injecting into either causes pain. The sheaths of the muscles contain pain fibers as does perineurium. The dura covering the optic sheath, the arterial and venous walls also contain pain fibers.

Sensationless placement of the needle in the mid-orbit is possible in awake patients once the needle passes through the skin or conjunctiva, which themselves can be blocked without producing pain. Pain means the needle is close to a structure that it shouldn't contact. The needle should be withdrawn, pressure applied, then the needle redirected.

Subsequent injection of anesthetic should be done with extreme caution. There may be a hole in the dura which will allow ingress of anesthetic into the subdural or subarachnoid spaces with resultant brain stem anesthesia.

The extraocular muscles contain stretch fibers. If anesthetic is injected at one milliliter per 10 seconds[34], the stretch fibers in the extraocular muscles are not activated and the orbit can be filled without generating pain, headache, nausea, vomiting, tachycardia or bradycardia. Fast filling can produce mania and cardiac arrest due to the oculocardiac reflex. Once total block of the stretch fibers is achieved, the eye can be moved about at will for strabismus surgery. A retrobulbar injection of 1 to 2 ml volume of anesthetic will almost never accomplish this as measured by Bosomworth.[63]

Arterial walls contain pain fibers. Ocular arteries are easily injured and can be entered by a needle within the muscle cone or in the orbital apex (as shown in Figure 1.10). The ophthalmic artery is most vulnerable where it branches into the central artery. There will be pain when this artery is touched unless the patient is sedated.

The tiny ciliary arteries and nerves are parallel to the optic nerve in central adipose spaces within septal compartments, and contain pain fibers. They can be injured if the needle approaches or passes the optic nerve at an acute angle as with a "retrobulbar needle aimed at the apex" or curved needle conal anesthetic techniques.

Ocular veins are located within the septal walls, except for the central retinal vein, which is within the dural sheath until its exit in the posterior orbit (as seen in Figure 1.32) about at the same area where the ophthalmic artery perforates the optic nerve to become the central artery. In this locus the vein is very vulnerable to injury. The superior orbital vein and inferior orbital vein are vulnerable in the deep orbit where septa anchor them to periosteum which has pain fibers.

Intravascular injection of anesthetic at a high rate carries great risk from misplaced needles because anesthetic can spread retrograde into the brain.[64] Injection at a rate of greater than 1 ml per 10 seconds in a properly placed needle in the mid-orbit causes pain,[34] probably by stretching proprioceptive fibers. Thus, slow injection rate to eliminate pain also minimizes danger of retrograde spread of anesthetic from intravascular injection, minimizes the cardiac depressant effects of the anesthetic if intravenous injection occurs, and minimizes the risk of inducing the oculocardiac reflex. Injection rate in the orbit should be no faster than 1 ml per 10 seconds; however many patients continue to survive injections at 10 times that rate.

When the conjunctiva is anesthetized with painless topical anesthetic[34] for transconjunctival blocks, or the skin for percutaneous blocks, it is possible to provide total anesthesia, globe akinesia, lid akinesia, and total autonomic block without producing pain: these patients enjoy totally pain-free anesthesia and surgery. The surgeon enjoys perfect operating conditions. That many surgeons expect less and patients accept it, is no reason for complacency.

Clinical Summary

The orbit is a unique structure for local anesthetic injection—it may be shallow or deep, it may have a generous or constricted opening, or contain a large or small globe which can be deep or shallow in the orbit. It may have tight or loose septal compartments, it has sympathetic nerves coursing within motor nerves instead of with the arteries and it is void of lymphatics. Because it is relatively easy to associate single injection of larger volumes of anesthetic placed deeper in the orbit with a higher incidence of good blocks, there is need for constraint on the part of the operator to provide maximal safety to persons with small orbits and tight septa.

Deep needle penetration into the posterior orbit increases the risk of injury and we agree with the recommendation that deep orbital or deep orbital apex blocks be done only with special blunted needles and with fluid injected ahead of the needle because of the packed, immobile state of the orbital apex.

Mid-orbital blocks through the avascular, atraumatic entrance sites down the adipose tissue compartments can be safely done with sharp block needles, if the anesthetist uses proper care and understands the anatomy and spatial relationships. Such blocks are uniformly safe and effective when individual variations in globe size, orbital length, and distance to the muscular cone are considered. Several injection sites are necessary in many orbits to provide anesthesia and akinesia from local anesthetic injection in the mid-orbit.

Remember, injection greater than one milliliter per ten seconds causes pain—inject no faster. This slow rate of injection will minimize the risk to the patient of inadvertent intravascular injection. Inject only as much anesthetic as the globe will tolerate without feeling tense or full. Knowing the anatomical structures of the orbit is key to placing needles safely into the orbit and injecting anesthetic with safety.

References

1. Koornneef L.: The first results of a new anatomical method of approach to the human orbit following a clinical enquiry. Acta Morphol Neerl Scand 12:259-282, 1974.
2. Koornneef L, Los JA: A new anatomical approach to the human orbit. Mod Probl Ophthalmol 14:49-56, 1975.
3. Koornneef L: The development of the connective tissue in the human orbit. Acta Morphol Neerl Scand 14:263-290, 1976.
4. Koornneef L: Details of the orbital connective tissue system in the adult. Acta Morphol Neerl Scand 15:1-34, 1977.
5. Koornneef L: The architecture of the musculo-fibrous apparatus in the human orbit. Acta Morphol Neerl Scand 15:35-64, 1977.
6. Koornneef L.: Spatial Aspects of Orbital Musculo-Fibrous Tissue in Man. Swets and Zeitlinger BV, Amsterdam and Lisse, 1977.
7. Zonneveld FW, Koornneef L, Hillen B, et al. Direct Multiplanar, High-resolution, Thin-section CT of the Orbit. Philips Medical Systems, Eindhoven, The Netherlands, 1984.
8. Zonneveld FW. Computed Tomography of the Temporal Bone and Orbit. Urban & Schwarzenberg, Baltimore, 1987.
9. Zonneveld FW, Koornneef L, Hillen B, de Slegte RG. Normal direct multiplanar CT anatomy of the orbit with correlative anatomic cryosections. Radiol Clin North Am. 25(3):381-407, May 1987.
10. de Jong RH. Physiology and Pharmacology of Local Anesthetics. Thomes, Springfield 1970. 114-36.
11. Koorneeff L: Sectional anatomy of the orbit. Aeolus Press, Amsterdam, 1981.
12. Koorneeff L: Orbital Connective Tissue. Chapter 32 of Biomedical Foundations of Ophthalmology, Thomas D. Duane. Harper & Row, Philadelphia, 1982.
13. Koornneef L. New insights in the human orbital connective tissue. Archiv Ophthal 1977; 95:1269-1273.
14. Koornneef L. Orbital Bony and Soft Tissue Anatomy. In: CA Gorman et al, eds. The Eye and Orbit in Thyroid Disease. New York: Raven Press, 1984:5-23.
15. Koornneef L. Eyelid and orbital fascial attachments and their clinical significance. Eye 1988;2:130-4.
16. Koornneef L, Mourtis M. Orbital decompression for decreased visual acuity or for cosmetic reasons. Orbit 7(4):225-38. Aeolus Press, Amsterdam, 1988.
17. Koornneef L, Schmidt ED, Van Der Gaag R. The Orbit: Structure, Autoantigens, and Pathology. In: Wall Jr, How J, eds. Hershman JM, series ed. Graves' Ophthalmopathy Current Issues in Endocrinology and Metabolism. Boston: Blackwell Scientific Publications, 1990:1-16.
18. Mourtis, MP, Koornneef L, Wiersinga WM, et al. Orbital decompression for Graves' ophthalmopathy by

inferomedial, by inferomedial plus lateral, and by coronal approach. Ophthalmology 97(5):638-41, May 1990.

19. Koornneef L, Zonneveld FW. The role of direct multiplanar high resolution CT in the assessment and management of orbital trauma. Radiol Clin North Am. 25(4):753-66, Jul 1987.

20. Parsons GS, Mathog RH. Orbital wall and volume relationships. Arch Otolargngol Head Neck Surg 1988:114;743-7.

21. Frazier-Byrne S. Personal Communication.

22. Katsev DA, Drews RC, Rose BT. An anatomic study of retrobulbar needle path length. Ophthalmology 1989:96;1221-4.

23. Atkinson WS. Anesthesia in Ophthalmology, First Edition. Charles C. Thomas, Springfield, 1955.

24. Atkinson WS. Anesthesia in Ophthalmology, Second Edition. Charles C. Thomas, Springfield, 1965.

25. Pautler SE, Grizzard WS, et al. Blindness from retrobulbar injection into the optic nerve. Ophth Surg 1986:17;334-7.

26. Unsold R, Stanley J, et al. The CT topography of retrobulbar anesthesia. Albrecht von Graefes Arch Klin Ophthalmol 1981:217;125-6.

27. Grizzard WS. Ophthalmic Anesthesia. In: Ophthalmology Annual. Ed. Reineche RD, RAven Press, New York, 1989.

28. Miller J. Functional anatomy of normal human rectus muscles. Vision Res 1989:29;223-40.

29. Foster AH, Carlson BM. Myotoxicity of local anesthetics and regeneration of the damaged muscle fibres. Anesth Analg 1980:59;727-35.

30. Rao V, Kawatra V. Ocular myotoxic effects of local anesthetics. Can J Ophthalmol 1988:23;171-3.

31. Rainin EA, Carlson BM. Postoperative diplopia and ptosis: a clinical hypothesis based on the myotoxicity of local anesthetics. Arch Ophthalmol 1985:103;1337-9.

32. Adriani J. Labat's Regional Anesthesia: Techniques and Clinical Applications, Fourth Edition. Warren H. Green, Inc., St. Louis, 1985.

33. Gifford H (Jr.). Motor block of extraocular muscles by deep orbital injection. Arch Ophthalmol 1949:41;5-19.

34. Gills JP, Loyd TL. A technique of retrobulbar block with paralysis of orbicularis oculi. Am Intraoc Implant Soc J 1983:9;339.

35. Johnson DE, Gills JP. Advanced Ophthalmic Anesthesia. Current Therapy in Ophthalmic Surgery, 1989.

36. Hamilton RC, Gimbel HV, Strunin L. Regional anesthesia for 12,000 cataract extractions and intraocular lens implantation procedures. Can J Anaesth 1988:35;615-23.

37. Knapp H. On cocaine and its use in ophthalmic and general surgery. Arch Ophthalmol 1884:13;402.

38. Braun HFW. Local Anesthesia. Lea & Febiger, Philadelphia, 1924, p 119.

39. Kelman C. Method suggested to reduce retrobulbar injection trauma. Ophthal Times, October 1, 1983.

40. Thornton S. Personal Communication.

41. Pitkin GP. Conduction Anesthesia. Eds: Southworth JL & Hingson RA. JB Lippincott Company, Philadelphia, 1946.

42. Pannu JS. Peribulbar vs. retrobulbar anesthetic techniques (letter). Ophthalmic Surg 1990:21;147-9.

43. Koziol J. Anatomy of the orbit. In: Principles and Practice of Ophthalmology. Eds: Peyman GA, Sanders DR, Goldberg MF. WB Saunders Company, Philadelphia, 1980.

44. Revised by RJ Last. Eugene Wolff's Anatomy of the Eye and Orbit, Fifth Edition. WB Saunders Company, Philadelphia, 1961.

45. Swan K. New drugs and techniques for ocular anesthesia. Amer Acad Ophthalmol & Otolaryngol 1956:60;368-75.

46. O'Brien CS. Local anesthesia. Arch Ophthalmol 1934:12;240.

47. Smith RB (ed). Anesthesia in Ophthalmology. Little, Brown and Company, Boston, 1973. International Ophthalmology Clinics, Summer 1973, 13(2).

47a. Linn JG, Smith RB. Intraoperative complications and their management. Smith RB (ed). Anesthesia in Ophthalmology. Little, Brown and Company, Boston, 1973. International Ophthalmology Clinics, Summer 1973, 13(2).

48a. Bloomberg L. Administration of periocular anesthesia. J Cataract Refract Surg 12:677-9;1986.

48b. Bloomberg L. Anterior periocular anesthesia: five years experience. J Cataract Refract Surg 17:508-11;1991.

49. Davis DB 2nd, Mandel MR. Peribulbar anesthesia (letter). J Cataract Refract Surg 1990:16;527-8.

50. Hill F. Personal Communication.

51. Drysdale DB. Experimental subdural retrobulbar injection of anesthetic. Ann Ophthalmol 1984:16;717-8.

52. Caramel JP, Bonnel F, Rabischong P. The oculomotor nerve: biometry and endoneural fascicular

systemization. Anat Clin 1983:5;159-68.

53. Nikki P, Ropo A, et al. Comparison of retrobulbar and periocular injection of lignocaine by computerised tomography. Brit J Ophthalmol 1991:75;417-20.

54. Vogl G, Schimek F, et al. Stereotactic retrobulbar anesthesia using CT. J Computer Assisted Tomography 1990:14;859-61.

55. Otto AJ, Spekreigse H. Volume discrepanicies in the orbit and the effect on the intra-orbital pressure: an experimental study in the monkey. Orbit 1989:8;233-44.

56. Duke-Elder Sir WS. Textbook of Ophthalmology, Volume 1. The C.V. Mosby Company, St. Louis, 1938.

57. Heerfordt GF. Uber das emphysem der orbita. Albrecht von Graefes, Archiv fur Ophtolmologie 1904:58;123-50.

58. Goldberg R, Marmor M, et al. Blindness following blepharoplasty: two case reports and a discussion of management. Ophthalmic Surg 1990:21;85-9.

59. McGetrick JJ, Wilson DG, et al. A search for lymphatic drainage of the monkey orbit. Arch Ophthalmol 1989:107;255-60.

60. Manson PN, Lazarus RB, et al. Pathways of sympathetic innervation to the superior and inferior (Muller's) tarsal muscles. Plast Reconst Surg 1986:78;33-40.

61. Gifford H Jr. A study of the vitreous pressure in cataract surgery. Tr Am Ophth Soc 1946:44;435-92.

62a. Hustead, RF. BSS takes the sting out of local anesthesia. Ocular Surgery News 4:39;Nov 1986.

62b. Hustead, RF. Patent #4938970.

63. Bosomworth PP, Ziegler CH, Jacoby J. The oculo-cardiac reflex in eye muscle surgery. Anesthesiology 1958:19;7-10.

64. Aldrete JA, Romo-Salas F, et al. Reverse arterial blood flow as a pathway for central nervous system toxic responses following injection of local anesthetics. Anesth Anal 1978:94;718-24.

65. Weiss J, Deichman C. A comparison of retrobulbar and periocular anesthesia for cataract surgery. Arch Ophthalmol 107:96-8;1989.

66. Bergen MP. Vascular Architechture in the Human Orbit. Swets & Zeitlinger B.V., Lisse, 1982.

67. Zahl K, Nassif, et al. Simulated Peribulbar Injection of Anesthetic. Ann Ophthalmol 1991:23;114-117.

68. Duverger. L'anesthésie locale en ophtalmologie. Masson et Cie, Paris, 1920.

69. Lowenstein A. Ueber regionare anasthesie in der orbita. Klin Monatsb f Augenh 592-601;1908.

Two

Robert F. Hustead, MD
Robert C. Hamilton, MB, BCh

PHARMACOLOGY

Background

This chapter discusses how anesthetic spreads from injection until the drug diffuses from nerve mantle to nerve core where interference with electrical conduction occurs. Concurrently, injectate is taken up from the vascular bed of the tissues to which it has spread and is redistributed systemically. The relationship of the volume and concentration of local anesthesic to the anesthesia or other effects it produces will be discussed.

Physicochemical principles and the laws of diffusion apply whether the drug is applied topically or injected; the unique chemical and physical characteristics of local anesthetic drugs that affect their motion through tears or tissues into nerve axons where they "block" the electrical propagation of the nerve impulse will be discussed. Current drugs will be analyzed to help the practitioner select the most effective.

Local anesthetics reversibly block peripheral and central nerve pathways when applied to or injected near nerves. They are intended to diffuse out of the nerve with no residual effects. The rare occurrence of irreversibility will be discussed.

Safety of the local anesthetics is measured by their reversible effect on nerves and lack of effect on other tissues, regardless of whether they are injected into the blood supply of the heart and brain.

Historical Perspective

The introduction of general anesthesia in 1846 was widely adopted. Patients wanted it for all operations by 1884, especially for those around the eye. However, general anesthesia was not welcomed by the ophthalmologist because it made the operation more difficult due to orbital congestion,[1] and the inordinate amount of time necessary for the patient "to be made ready."[2] Additionally, the proximity of the anesthetist, trying to keep the patient breathing and motionless made for an uncomfortable mess.[1-3] Besides, general anesthesia carried the risk of death.

Koller's pioneering demonstration in 1884[1,4,5] of the effect of local anesthesia for ophthalmic surgery was done using topical cocaine which abolished pain even though it did not keep the lids and the eye immobile. The surgeon/anesthetist applying cocaine could do surgery more skillfully, with little or no pain. He could expect better results than the conventional surgeon using an anesthetist and general anesthesia, hypnosis, or no anesthesia at all, providing the patient was cooperative.

Injection of cocaine in the orbit to provide akinesia of the globe and freedom from pain of deeper structures was the logical extension of the surgeon/anesthetist's skill. Such injections followed within weeks of the report of Koller's discovery of the topical effectiveness of cocaine. The concept of conduction anesthesia with local anesthetic drugs to block conduction of the nerve impulse to produce anesthesia and akinesia was established. Cocaine was praised because it caused relatively little pain on injection, was a potent vasoconstrictor, and blocked sensory and motor nerves making for cleaner operations and better surgical results.

Orbital injection techniques were only gradually accepted because of the toxicity of cocaine (often due to impurities), its cost, ineffectiveness, blindness and death reports from intraorbital injection in the apex of the orbit or posterior to the ethmoid nerve. Injection to block the ciliary ganglion was reserved for enucleation or extraction of the globe.[2,3,6,7]

Better surgical conditions could be obtained by topically applying cocaine or infiltrating small amounts in the area to be cut rather than injecting the same volume of anesthetic in the orbit. Orbital injection often caused uncomfortable side effects such as syncope, cold sweats, and hallucinations, which were rare with topical administration or local infiltration. In the first published reports of cocaine use in the United States, Knapp reported such effects with 6 minims (0.37 ml) of 2% cocaine for enucleation and warned of the possibility of death.[1]

Certain clinical concepts of cocaine use for surgery to preserve vision, e.g. cataract and glaucoma surgery, were established based on the early observation of cocaine's pharmacologic effects, especially its short duration and toxic attributes. They included:

- Anesthetization of the globe performed by the surgeon in the operating room after preparation of the surgical field to ensure the operation be accomplished with minimum waste of precious anesthesia time.
- The sparing use of local anesthesia which leads to epithelial sloughing of the cornea.
- Large injected volumes cause toxic reactions and poor surgical conditions such as vitreous prolapse or expulsive hemorrhage, therefore only small volumes of local anesthetic should be injected in the orbit.
- Avoidance of massage or pressure on the globe after the block which leads to a soft eye and difficult lens delivery.
- Good surgical conditions can be obtained with topical administration on the cornea preceded or followed by small injections in the medial and lateral orbit (orbital blocks) or subconjunctival injection at the limbus extended along the muscles, plus additional topical whenever the patient has pain.
- Avoidance of deep orbital or ciliary ganglion blocks except for enucleation.
- Maximizing the use of sedatives to minimize the amount of local anesthetic required.
- Encouragement for the search for more effective, longer lasting, less toxic local anesthetic drugs.

Because cocaine worked even better for the ophthalmologist when the new drug epinephrine was added, the search for an "ideal" ophthalmic local anesthetic gained little momentum. Epinephrine extended useful anesthesia time, decreased vitreous pressure, bleeding, and the amount of cocaine needed. Most eye surgery did not require dangerously large amounts of cocaine, and cocaine worked faster, dilated the pupil better, controlled bleeding better, and hurt no more topically or upon injection than other drugs.

Furthermore, the new oral sedatives made cocaine anesthesia even more convenient. Sedation was supposed to make cocaine less toxic and more effective—and the patient more comfortable and compliant.

Safer local anesthetic drugs replaced cocaine for general surgical use, the safest of which was procaine. But procaine only gradually replaced cocaine in ophthalmology because of cocaine's efficiency, clinical advantage, and familiarity; it was still the anesthetic of choice for subconjunctival injection by O'Brien as late as 1934.[8] Topical cocaine gradually gave way to butyn and tetracaine.

Procaine eventually became the standard for injection in ophthalmology, in part because it had fewer undesirable autonomic and cerebral effects and was not addicting, but primarily because procaine was more stable in solution, had a longer shelf life, and could be purchased in bottles ready for use, whereas cocaine had to be prepared daily. Furthermore, procaine was far less expensive and free from the potential for drug abuse.

However, the clinical concepts of local anesthesia for eye surgery based on the early pharmacologic observations of cocaine delayed more rational pharmacologic considerations with procaine. That the orbit is a closed hydraulic space also delayed further development.

Substituting procaine for cocaine appeared to have little pharmacologic benefit and the established clinical concepts of cocaine use were reinforced with the addition of a block of the facial nerve or eye lids to prevent squinting or lid squeezing during cataract surgery. Topical application of tetracaine 1% and subconjunctival injection of small doses of anesthetic (less than 1 ml of 2-4% procaine) were used. O'Brien, as late as 1928, recommended 0.3 ml of cocaine 4% mixed equally with 1:1,000 epinephrine at 12:00 to anesthetize the conjunctiva and iris.[8]

Minimal doses of procaine were injected because sudden death was feared and because larger injections elevated intraocular pressure. Procaine was rapidly removed from the orbit and the block was short acting unless combined with epinephrine. The added epinephrine decreased intraocular pressure, and therefore was added in 1:3,000 to 1:5,000 concentrations. Many persons exhibited toxic reactions to procaine/epinephrine when it was injected in the orbit in any but the smallest quantity. Larger quantities could cause syncope and cold sweats similar to those seen with cocaine. Physicians were concerned that larger amounts could cause death.

Anesthesia with small amounts of procaine and lidocaine would have remained the techniques of choice for cataract surgery until today if not for Atkinson's report in 1949 that larger injections of local anesthetic to produce akinesia were feasible with hyaluronidase. The volume of anesthetic could also be increased considerably without causing more than a temporary increase in intraocular pressure. This rise could be eliminated by massaging the globe to spread the anesthetic and facilitate absorption of the hyaluronidase/local anesthetic solution. He continued to encourage injection in the cone instead of the apex. His recommended dosage of 2% procaine in the muscle cone for cataract surgery rose from 1 ml in 1934[9] to 1-1.5 ml in 1948.[10] After hyaluronidase was purified and available for routine use, dosage stabilized at an amount that produced noticeable proptosis (2 to 3 ml) in 1955,[11] and 4 to 8 ml in 1964.[12] He conservatively recommended in the second edition of his book in 1965, a volume of "3 ml or more in the average orbit."[13]

The reliability, safety, and efficacy of the larger dosage of procaine/hyaluronidase mixture for cone injection was well accepted when it was noted that lidocaine solution, which had been recently introduced into the American market, spread better than procaine[14] even though it seemed to be more painful on injection.[15] Cataract patients rarely complained of injection pain though, because the sedatives induced amnesia. Painful memory was often ascribed to the "resistance" of the patient—an indication for general anesthesia for future surgery.

The combination of hyaluronidase, larger anesthetic volume, and prolonged, deliberate pressure over the orbit was shown by Kirsch[16] to produce the hypotony of the globe necessary for ideal intracapsular cataract extraction conditions. This hypotony by oculocompression with reduction of vitreous volume allowed the conditions necessary to operate well despite the early fear that a soft eye created problems in lens extraction. The soft eye and vitreous dehydration allowed space for intraocular lens implantation, which soon followed.

However, lidocaine did not last long enough for the more time consuming extracapsular surgery with lens implantation, so the longer lasting mepivacaine gained popularity as did tetracaine.[17] Bupivacaine was added to lidocaine[18] or mepivacaine.[19] These drugs caused much more pain on injection than lidocaine or procaine.

The long acting bupivacaine, newly released from the European markets, had less spreading effect and much slower onset than lidocaine, which became an incentive to add even greater volumes of total solution. Volumes of 5 ml of lidocaine/bupivacaine were becoming standard in much the same way that large volumes of lidocaine were popularized.[12] Lidocaine/bupivacaine provided longer blocks and postoperative analgesia, which patients appreciated. Etidocaine appeared next and worked as fast as lidocaine and lasted as long as bupivacaine.[20]

The search for an ideal local anesthetic seemed to be answered by etidocaine or lidocaine/mepivacaine/bupivacaine mixtures despite the warnings of textbook authors who suggested that mixtures were not indicated.[21]

However, incomplete akinesia of the extraocular muscles was not rare with the new mixtures, as had also been true with cone injections of even 8% procaine or 4% lidocaine. This variability of obtaining ocular akinesia from injection had always been an inconvenience, but physicians were more concerned about vitreous loss in a moving eye. Now this could be solved more conveniently by adding bupivacaine or etidocaine. Reduced vitreous loss meant better vision; better vision meant more patients. Bupivacaine and etidocaine lasted so long that two patients could be blocked and the globe massaged to reduce intraocular pressure. Whichever patient had the best ocular akinesia went to surgery first and the second was given a supplemental injection expected to produce 100% akinesia.

A third patient could then be prepared for block. This worked well in some teaching hospitals where the residents blocked for the staff in another operating room, or in a group where one associate was willing to block for another. It was even better for operating room efficiency when the hospital allowed blocks in an area outside of the operating room.

Blocking outside the operating room was a totally new concept in many private hospitals because it was always considered mandatory for surgeons to block their own patients in the operating room. The block and 10 minutes of digital ocular massage were considered part of the operating room time, which was billed at $200/hour, increasing revenue but not operating room efficiency.

The ambulatory surgery facility was designed so that the anesthetist blocked the next patient or had a second anesthesia provider do it. That way the anesthetist could prepare one patient for surgery while the surgeon was completing the first procedure or could have two blocked ahead of time for safety.

Rapid turnover was therefore assured with no down time for the operating room or the surgeon. Cataract surgery smoothly increased from 250,000 in 1967 to 1,300,000 in 1990.

This situation produced ideal operating conditions for many surgeons whose patients were pain-free and with long lasting blocks. Many surgeons thought outpatient cataract surgery was in the patient's best interest.

The move to outpatient surgery encouraged the use of less sedation. Long lasting oral or intramuscular sedatives interfered with early ambulation and required additional attendants. The patient needed a short, rapid acting sedative for the block because that was the only painful part of the procedure when the ensuing block was perfect.

The block, ophthalmologists realized, could be made less painful by utilizing painless or almost painless topical anesthetics and injectable local anesthetics,[22] eliminating the orbicularis block,[23] and slow injection of body temperature anesthetic solution. With such techniques sedation could be minimized or eliminated for most patients.

It was becoming easier to diagnose the poor and the perfect blocks because patients were alert when unsedated. Akinesia and anesthesia could be checked before surgery to ensure a pain-free operating room experience.

When a block was perfect, the patient felt no discomfort and experienced six to 24 hours of post-operative analgesia. If the block wasn't perfect patients would complain, move, and remember this discomfort because minimal sedation was used. Such a situation became a strong incentive to increase the volume of anesthetic mixture and introduce needles deeper into the orbit. Apnea and blindness resulted.

Injections deep in the apex had been known for 100 years to cause blindness. Injections outside the muscle cone in the retrobulbar space or periorbital space (peribulbar[24] or periocular[25]), shallow in the cone with the eyes ahead,[26] or lateral in the cone with the eyes up[19] were used to improve safety. All these techniques required larger volume injection for effectiveness than the Atkinson conal technique or the apical Gifford technique, but placed needles further from the optic nerve.

Patients who stopped breathing three to ten minutes after their blocks were reported. This brainstem anesthesia was blamed on bupivacaine until the problem was seen with lidocaine/bupivacaine mixtures or lidocaine alone. Also, it was more frequent with larger single volume of injection and longer needles. Since no cases of death were reported in more than 50 episodes because of the timely intervention of anesthesia providers, the role of that provider became further entrenched. Brain stem anesthesia from subdural or subarachnoid spread was an established syndrome. Would placing the needle further from the optic nerve solve the problem or would volume of injection have to be curtailed?

Anesthesia providers began to tabulate data on volume of anesthetic and locus of injection to eliminate blindness and apnea, without diminishing effectiveness.

Five known factors were investigated during the past two decades—changing anesthetic drug, increasing the concentration of local anesthetic, changing concentration of hyaluronidase, adding epinephrine to the block solution, and changing the pH of the injected anesthetic solution.

Studies showed that akinesia could be improved by using 4% lidocaine instead of 4% procaine,[14] using 8% procaine instead of 4% procaine,[27] using of 4% lidocaine instead of 2%,[14] using lidocaine alone instead of adding bupivacaine, using bupivacaine alone in 0.75% concentration instead of 0.5%,[19] adding hyaluronidase,[28,29] by adding epinephrine if hyaluronidase was used,[30] and increasing the pH of the solution by adding sodium bicarbonate ($NaHCO_3$).[31]

But none of these manipulations changed the fact that some patients would have an incomplete block from one or even two 3 to 10 ml injections of anesthetic in the "safe areas" of the orbit. Incomplete injection occurred with the cone injection of Atkinson, the lateral cone block of Gills/Loyd, the deep peribulbar sites of Davis, the shallow peribulbar sites of Wang,[32] or the periocular sites of Bloomberg.[25]

Between three to 20% of patients needed additional injections in one, two or three sites to provide complete akinesia. So the optimum site for supplementary injection was sought to provide total akinesia with safety.

The addition of hyaluronidase only slightly decreased the incidence of incomplete blocks, but was deemed essential in the rapid removal of fluid from the orbit and to decrease vitreous volume in these large volume injection techniques for cataract surgery. For retinal detachment and enucleation, it seemed the additional volume provided better surgical conditions.

Meanwhile, surgical technique for cataract surgery was changing from extracapsular with 7 mm lens implantation to small incision phacoemulsification and small profile lenses. Some surgeons believed that the marked hypotony produced by oculocompression, thought to be necessary in the days of extracapsular cataract surgery, was no longer indicated, and some reported that ocular motility was acceptable even during phacoemulsification, although others thought slight movement led to compromise of the endothelium or the posterior capsule.

There are surgeons/anesthetists and anesthesia providers who would like to offer optimal anesthesia conditions with optimal safety to assure that the operative result was not compromised by inadequate anesthesia conditions.

Optimum surgical anesthesia requires knowledge of:

- How to avoid pain with local anesthetic drug injection and the benefits to the patients;
- How local anesthetics can penetrate nerves more effectively and where this process compromises safety;
- How to select agents that wear off quickly for procedures requiring no post-op analgesia and quick return of function;
- How to improve the safety of local anesthetics to nerves and the rest of the body;
- How to extend post-operative analgesia with local anesthetics and its benefit to the patient;
- How sedatives make local anesthetics safer or more effective;
- The possibility of safer and less painful local anesthetic drugs in the future.

Pharmacologic advances of local anesthetic drugs is thoroughly discussed in several current and up-to-date texts and review articles. This chapter will not concentrate on reviewing those aspects, which are esoteric to the scientist. The most extensive current book on this matter, *Neural Blockade in Clinical Anesthesia in Management of Pain,* by Cousins and Bridenbaugh, published by Lippencott and the review in *Anesthesiology* 1990:72;711-34 by Butterworth and Strichartz are excellent sources. These writings, with extensive bibliography, handle such matters well, even though they only briefly mention the use of these drugs in ophthalmology.

The treatises in the pharmacology of local anesthetics in older ophthalmology texts has been lacking in scientific or clinical understanding of mode of action, side-effects, or the toxicity of the local anesthetic drugs because they borrowed too heavily from scientific sources or anesthesiology texts and ignored the specific problems of the ophthalmic use of these drugs.

The treatment of local anesthetics for ophthalmic use in anesthesiology text books and reviews is poor because few anesthesiologists have spent time clinically or in research in the area of ophthalmic regional anesthesia. The anatomical differences between the brachial plexus and the epidural space on the one hand, and the orbit on the other hand, have been slow to attract attention.

Pharmacology of Local Anesthetics

Chemistry

Table 2.1 shows the physicochemical profile of anesthetic drugs commonly used in ophthalmology. All clinically useful local anesthetics are tertiary amines separated by a bridge of ester or amide linkage of six to nine Angstroms from an unsaturated ring (aromatic and usually benzene).

- Hydrophilic alkyl or aromatic amino group;
- Lipophilic aromatic residue;
- A linkage group which is either an ester or an amide.

The tertiary amine is a proton acceptor and bears a positive charge in aqueous solution giving that end of the molecule a hydrophilic character. The aromatic end is lipophilic. The potency, onset time, duration of action, and selectivity are influenced by the chemical configuration of the two ends of this molecule. The linkage gives rise to two major groups of effective local anesthetics—the ester group and the amide group.

Procaine is the prototype ester local anesthetic and lidocaine is considered the prototype amide, although procainamide or Pronestyl® was actually synthesized many years before lidocaine.

Procaine has a first-cousin, tetracaine (Pontocaine®); lidocaine has a first-cousin, etidocaine; and mepivacaine has a first-cousin, bupivacaine. The cousins have additional side chains that change the chemical characteristics and lead to very long local anesthetic action and cardiovascular toxicity.

Cocaine, bupivacaine, and mepivacaine are racemic mixtures. The differential selectivity of stereo-isomers is being investigated with renewed interest.

The safety of the dextro-isomer of cocaine was established in 1924,[33] but it never caught on in commercial use, largely because its production was more expensive than procaine. It was supposedly an excellent anesthetic, free of cardiotoxic effects and non-addicting[34]—but so was procaine.

The new drug, Ropivacaine® is a racemic mixture, but will be marketed as the levo (S)-isomer, which has been shown to be a very effective local anesthetic and has much less cardiovascular toxicity than does the dextro (R)-isomer, which has less anesthetic duration and more cardiovascular toxicity. Ropivacaine® is entering clinical trials and may well be the answer for a long lasting local anesthetic drug with less cardiac toxicity.

Agent	Chemical Configuration: Aromatic Lipophilic	Intermediate Chain	Amine Hydrophilic	Mol. Wt. (1)	H₂O Solubility pH 7.4, 37°C (2)	Lipid Solubility (3)	Protein Binding (4)	pKa at 37°C (25°C) (5)	% Base pH 7.4 (6)	Available Conc. % (7)	pH (8)	NaHCO₃ to pH 7.3 (9)	Equi-Conc. % (10)	Relative Onset (11)	Duration Hours (12)	Max Dose (13)
ESTERS																
Cocaine	(benzene ring)	H₂COOC—CH—CH—CH₂ / CO—O—CH—CH—N—CH₃ / CH₂—CH—CH₂		303	4		yes	8.8 (8.4)		2T 4T 10T				S	1/3T	2
Procaine Novocaine	H₂N—(benzene)	COOCH₂CH₂	N(C₂H₅)(C₂H₅)	236	20–48	1	5	8.7 (8.9)	3	0.5 1 2 4			2	M	1/2 3/4 1	10
Tetracaine Pontocaine	H₂N—(benzene)	COOCH₂CH₂	N(CH₃)(CH₃)	264	1.4	80	85	(8.46)	7	0.25 0.5 1T 2T				S	1–2 2–3	2
Proparacaine Ophthane Ophthetic Alcaine	H₂N—(benzene)	COOCH₂CH₂	N(C₂H₅)(C₂H₅)	294	?					0.5T				F	1/3	?
Benoxinate Dorsacaine	H₂N—(benzene)	COOCH₂CH₂	N(C₂H₅)(C₂H₅)	307	?					0.4T				F	1/4	?
AMIDES																
Lidocaine Xylocaine Ultracaine	(benzene) CH₃ CH₃	NHCOCH₂	N(C₂H₅)(C₂H₅)	234	24	4	65	7.7 (7.9)	25	0.5 1 2,4 4T 20	6.5 +/-	1 1 1,? ?	2.0	S M F F Dil	1/2 3/4 1 1–2 Dil	6
Etidocaine Duranest	(benzene) CH₃ CH₃	NHCOCH (C₂H₅)	N(C₂H₅)(C₃H₇)	276	?	140	95	(7.7)	33	.5 1 1.5	4	ppt above 6.5	1	M F F	1–2 2–3 2–4	3
Mepivacaine Carbocaine Polocaine	(benzene) CH₃	NHCO	CH₃—N (ring)	246	15	1	74	7.6 (7.7)	39	1 2 3	5.5	1 1 0.6	1.5	M F F	1 1 1 1/2	6
Bupivacaine Marcaine Sensorcaine	(benzene) CH₃ CH₃	NHCO	C₄H₉—N (ring)	288	0.83	30	95	8.1 (8.16)	15	0.25 0.5 0.75	4.5 to 6	0.1 0.1 0.05 to pH 6.9	0.5	S M F	1 1–3 2–4	2
Ropivacaine	(benzene) CH₃	NHCO	N—C₃H₇ (ring)	274		2.8	90–95	(8.1)		Expt	?	?	0.75	?	?	?

All the clinically useful local anesthetics are insoluble in water and relatively unstable in their base amine form. However, all form salts with the organic acids. Solutions of the organic salt in water are stable and can be autoclaved for sterilization. The amide drugs withstand repeated autoclaving, causing no decrease in potency if the pH of solution is between 3 and 6.5. Stability is less true for the esters, which gradually lose potency with repeated autoclaving, especially tetracaine. These drugs become less stable as the pH is raised. Therefore, they are bottled with a pH less than 6.5 for prolonged shelf life. The ionization constant of the water solution of the acid salt can be measured. When the concentration of the protonated form (acid salt) equals the base form, the chemical constant pK_a is established (table one). The amount of base form at normal pH of 7.4 is also given in table one.

Alkalinization of the acid solution of these salts causes precipitation whenever the solubility of the base amine form is exceeded. This point is pH, concentration, and temperature dependent. Procaine and lidocaine form a temporary cloudiness with gradual precipitation. Mepivacaine will precipitate fairly rapidly and adhere to the walls of the syringe and needle at pH 7.2 and 2% concentration; bupivacaine and etidocaine will rapidly form a gummy mass below a pH of 6.9 in concentrations exceeding 0.25%.

Injection into tissue and tissue fluids immediately decreases the effective concentration of the local anesthetics as the substance partitions between cells and fluids. The higher the lipid solubility, the more likely the molecule will enter cells; the higher the water solubility, the more will enter plasma and attach to proteins or lipoproteins. This is why the amide group of drugs tend to spread better in tissues than do the esters and why it was thought necessary to inject the ester group of drugs closer to their target organ for clinical effectiveness. Procaine injected in larger volumes and higher concentration would probably spread as well as lidocaine, but would have exaggerated tissue and body toxicity.

The ester linkage is readily broken down in the body in a very rapid reaction with plasma cholinesterase and in a slower reaction with tissue cholinesterase. When an ester is injected around a nerve, the anesthetic diffuses from the injection site towards the nerve in contact with body fluids and tissue. Body fluids breakdown the ester local anesthetic molecule to inactive products so that as diffusion continues, the concentration head is diminished more rapidly than with molecules of the amides not broken down during the diffusion process.

Procaine owes its safety to rapid plasma breakdown of the ester linkage by plasma cholinesterase. The procaine molecule has great cardiac toxicity with a narrow therapeutic window in the absence of plasma or tissue esterases, as do most all ester local anesthetics. This is a great disadvantage in the use of ester locals because certain persons have low or absent plasma cholinesterase, estimated from 1:4,000-1:10,000. Such persons may have a lethal cardiac response to the ester local anesthetic drugs from rapid topical

Table 2.1 (see facing page)
Footnotes for the columns in Table:
*—Chiral Carbon, Racemic; 2—mg salt per ml H_2O at 37°C; 3—mg salt per ml olive oil at 37°C; 7—commercial solutions with and without preservations are available and with or without epinephrine; 8—all solutions with epinephrine, pH 3-4; 9—approximate 1990—manufacturer's may change pH without notice and pH decreases with shelf life; 11—relativity is quite variable; 12—duration is approximate and quite variable. Duration is increased by use of epinephrine or repeat injections. Topical is for 2 qtts (longer if more qtts are used).; 13—assumed no intravenous injection and that injection is done slowly.

absorption, tissue absorption, or intravenous injection of normal or much lower than normal amounts. Thus, procaine shares with cocaine the reputation of causing unexplained death.

The ester group of drugs, *except proparacaine,* are hydrolyzed by esterases to para-aminobenzoic acid, which attaches as a ligand to many proteins, and is thought to be highly allergenic. Methylparaben and proparaben, which are added to multi-dose vials of ester or amide local anesthetics as bacteriostatic or bacteriocidal drugs, contain para-aminobenzoic acid or benzoic acid nuclei and have the same allergenic potential. Therefore, multi-dose vials of amide should not be used in patients suspected of ester allergy.

Because of these two disadvantages, the ester local anesthetics should have little place in modern pharmacology, and would have none, except as topical anesthetics in ophthalmology.

Safe clinical use of the esters benoxinate and tetracaine in ophthalmology requires that they be used in the lowest possible dosage to avoid lethal reactions in those with unsuspected low cholinesterase activity or allergy to the para-aminobenzoic moieties. They should not be used in large quantities or in quantities that will be absorbed through the nasal-lacrimal apparatus or mucous membranes. In these circumstances topical amides should be substituted. All the amides are effective in the proper concentration and at proper pH.

The clinical use of proparacaine for topical application on the cornea has greater merit. It is not a para-aminobenzoic acid ester and can be used as a painless topical anesthetic solution.

The amide group of drugs are not broken down in the tissues locally or in the bloodstream, with the exception of prilocaine. Unfortunately, prilocaine induces methemoglobin formation in the bloodstream and, therefore, is believed to be less than an ideal agent.

Metabolism of the remaining amide group of drugs takes place primarily in the liver. The distribution volumes and half-life of the amide drugs have been extensively studied, especially that lidocaine, which is extensively used in ambulances, emergency rooms, and coronary care units for cardiac arrhythmias.

Commercial Formulation
of Local Anesthetic Solutions

Painful and Non-Painful Solution Preparation

All commercial local anesthetics are bottled in class I glass or plastic containers as isotonic solutions in water or sodium chloride solution (sodium/calcium chloride solution for mepivacaine) and pH adjusted for optimal shelf life.

The addition of methylparaben and proparaben to anesthetic solutions manufactured in the United States is very common and are bottled in multi-use vials. These allergenic and neurotoxic substances are poor at maintaining sterility. In fact, proparaben is known as a substrate for some fungi.

Therefore, multi-use vials should not be considered sterile once opened and should be used with great caution. Tetracaine is bacteriostatic to many bacteria in ordinary concentrations and inhibits the growth of many bacteria. However, the literature is very incomplete on its spectrum and that of the other local anesthetics. Their bacteriocidal/viricidal quality is unreliable.

All local anesthetics can be transfilled into currently available plastic and glass syringes. When performed under sterile conditions, the drug remains stable for long periods and no interaction has been shown with the plasticizers or the rubber of disposable syringes. However, no manufacturer has published guidelines establishing how long these solutions can be stored, and the United States Pharmacopeia (USP) addresses the problem in the generic transfer section. Therefore, most pharmacists discourage using local anesthetics that have been stored in glass or plastic syringes for longer than 24 hours unless refrigerated, and then refrigerated for only 48 hours. It is not known how long they can be stored.

Ampules or vials with epinephrine have 0.1% sodium metabisulfite added as an anti-oxidant and are bottled at a pH of 3 to 3.5 to prevent the epinephrine from oxidizing. Sodium metabisulfite is allergenic to many persons with asthma and can cause respiratory failure. Sodium metabisulfite is also thought to be neurotoxic and should not be injected in the orbit, in the authors' opinion.

The vast majority of local anesthetics for topical or regional anesthesia use are lidocaine, mepivacaine, and bupivacaine, and the topical anesthetics lidocaine, proparacaine, benoxinate, or tetracaine. Tetracaine and benoxinate may be eliminated because of their allergenicity and lethality with cholinesterase deficiency. Proparacaine and the amides are appropriate substitutes.

Considerable research was done trying to establish optimal solutions for anesthetic use; hypertonic and hypotonic were extensively studied. Many have clinical advantages over isotonic solutions under certain circumstances. Nonetheless, the USP requires all to be distributed as isotonic solutions unless they are diluted before use, such as 20% lidocaine for intravenous use in coronary care units.

Most useful local anesthetics form an isotonic solution with water in approximately a 4% concentration. Therefore, 4% procaine and 4% lidocaine solutions are bottled in water. Distilled water is one of the most painful substances that can be injected. Solutions of procaine and lidocaine in 4% concentrations are very painful on injection. Whether the pain is entirely due to the absence of sodium and chloride or the high concentration of anesthetic and hydrogen ion remains to be investigated.

When local anesthetics are bottled in concentrations less than 4%, sodium chloride or other salts are added to make an isotonic solution—roughly 3.3% sodium chloride for a 3% solution, 0.45% sodium chloride for a 2% solution, 0.65% for a 1% solution, 0.75% for a 0.5% solution, and 0.8% for a 0.25% solution. The pH of those solutions bottled without epinephrine is between 5 and 7, and usually none are bottled above a pH of 6.6 (see Table 2.1).

The high hydrogen ion concentration (low pH) of these solutions causes pain on injection. For a given pH, all produce pain, with, in ascending order, procaine causing the least, then lidocaine,[15] bupivacaine, and etidocaine. All of these local anesthetics, except bupivacaine and etidocaine, could be bottled at a pH approaching the physiologic normal of 7.2 to 7.4, although their shelf lives would be shortened.

Addition of sodium bicarbonate to the commercial acid solutions to reduce pain has been recommended. It effectively relieves the sharp burning pain, changing an injection from very uncomfortable to quite tolerable for most individuals.[35,36,37] The addition of 1 ml of $NaHCO_3$ (8.4%) to 10 ml lidocaine or carbocaine is recommended to reduce pain.

One percent solutions of local anesthetic are available with approximately 0.65% sodium chloride. The sodium and chloride ionic strength do not induce pain if the pH is raised above 7. This can be done with sodium bicarbonate, sodium citrate, or sodium acetate. The 2% solution of lidocaine and procaine can also be buffered to 7.4 without precipitation and is relatively painless, however, 2% mepivacaine gradually precipitates above 7.1 and plugs needles.

One percent carbocaine, 1% lidocaine, and 1% procaine solutions can be pH adjusted to above 7 and produce minimal pain on injection. Carbocaine 1% begins to precipitate at approximately a pH of 7.3, but lidocaine and procaine do not precipitate at 7.6. Both are forgiving of overly zealous efforts to raise the pH above 6.9, which appears critical to eliminate the burning pain of injection. Etidocaine and bupivacaine are very painful on injection. Etidocaine cannot be pH adjusted into a range that approaches the pH of normal tissues; it forms a gummy mass at at 0.05% at pH 6.5. Bupivacaine precipitates or forms a gummy mass only above a concentration of 0.05% at a pH of 7.0, and therefore can be injected painlessly. It is much more effective than one might think and has very rapid onset time.

It has been recommended that 1 ml of 8.4% sodium bicarbonate solution be added to 1% or 2% local anesthetic solutions at injection to eliminate or reduce pain. However, this concentration of sodium ion added to normal saline will induce an aching pain of its own. Sodium ion and chloride ion much above or below plasma levels will also induce pain.[37,38] Therefore, one needs to be very careful of the amount of bicarbonate added to specific solutions if the object is to eliminate pain.

Alkalinizing local anesthetic solutions began in the recent era with the observations of Gros and Ritchie that alkalinization should improve onset time and increase potency.[39,40] The reduction of pain was fortunate. Unfortunately, different batches of local anesthetic have different amounts of hydrogen ion added in manufacturing, and thus one needs to correlate the clinical effect with the amount of bicarbonate added and/or use a pH meter to raise the pH above 7, and keep the sodium and chloride concentrations out of pain inducing range.

All electrolyte solutions cause pain when injected in the dermis at a pH of less than 7.0, except 0.90% NaCl .9% benzyl alcohol,[15] or when the sodium and chloride concentrations are widely disparate from that found in normal plasma. All the commercial local anesthetics cause pain on injection. Home-made solutions of 0.5-2% procaine and lidocaine in balanced salt solution at pH 7.2-7.4 are painless according to Hustead's experience.

All local anesthetic molecules induce pain if they are applied on or close to nerves when the concentration is beyond a certain point, even though the pH, Na+, and Cl- are within the physiologic range.

If the concentration of local anesthetic is below that threshold concentration, it can be applied or injected and cause no pain, but if it is too dilute it will not produce anesthesia. To make a local anesthetic solution painless, the pH must be above 7, the concentration of active local anesthetic molecules must be below the threshold to induce pain at that pH, and the solutions must be controlled for sodium chloride and other organic cations and anions, some of which elicit pain in dilute amounts, i.e., lactate, gluconate, borate, sulphate, and phosphate.

Very dilute solutions of all the commercial anesthetics, except etidocaine, can be prepared by dilution with balanced salt solution (BSS of various manufacturer). The resultant mixture is almost painless on injection, yet quite effective therapeutically. The advantage of Alcon BSS® no longer exists since its sodium of 155 and pH of 7.0 are in the range of other manufacturers. Prior to 1988, Alcon BSS® had a pH of 7.8, Na+ 140, and Cl- 108 and made an ideal diluent for commercial anesthetics.

The pharmacist or the physician can transfer local anesthetics into balanced salt solution under sterile conditions, withdraw the dilute anesthetic mixture and store it in glass or plastic syringes for use. Such techniques are used daily to produce other sterile injectable drugs in the pharmacy of most hospitals. A 1:10 dilution of all the currently known anesthetics makes a useful, almost painless local anesthetic solution. Prepared and stored aseptically at 4°C, the solutions are stable for over six months. The dilute solutions are effective for starting IVs and infiltration of the skin and connective tissue before regional blocks; they are quite painless at 35°C.

Bacteriostatic saline (0.9% NaCl 0.9% benzyl alcohol) is not recommended for nerve block because the anesthetic effect is so short and the solution is neurotoxic.[41]

Topical Anesthetic Formulation

Tetracaine is the only topical anesthetic that is prepared for single use without preservatives in a dropper bottle. Proparacaine and benoxinate contain the bacteriocide, benzalkonium chloride, which effectively destroys the lipid and mucous layers of the tear film, thereby allowing the molecules direct access to the corneal nerve endings.

All amide and ester local anesthetics are made even more effective topically if the pH is adjusted to the alkaline 7.6-7.8 of tears. Lidocaine is especially effective at that pH in a concentration of 4%.

All the topical anesthetic formulations burn upon application to the cornea. The amount of stinging and burning varies with different persons and different drugs. Some individuals are more sensitive to tetracaine than proparacaine and vice versa. However, usually only the first drop burns and stings. If the first drop has adequate contact time with the tear film, it produces sufficient anesthetization so that the subsequent drops usually do not hurt. The first drop can produce intense lid spasm and may have led to further damage of already compromised eyes in emergency rooms. This first drop should be diluted and pH adjusted to reduce pain, especially for children and patients with wounded eyes.

A dilute, painless topical anesthetic can be prepared by the dilution of one part of proparacaine 0.5% solution into 15 ml of balanced salt solution. This solution is stable for about six weeks at room temperature and three months if refrigerated. It should be kept out of the light as much as possible. The solution does not contain a bacteriocidal agent in effective concentration and should be used cautiously to avoid contamination.

The author has been unable to prepare painless, effective topical solutions of tetracaine, benoxinate, lidocaine, mepivacaine, or bupivacaine. The 0.25% lidocaine solution in BSS, however, causes only slight pain of short duration when a drop is instilled in the conjunctival sac; it takes four drops for 0.25% lidocaine to be painless after which it is possible to instill 4% lidocaine and produce topical anesthesia similar to that obtained with cocaine. pH adjustment of 4% lidocaine makes it more effective, as mentioned earlier.

However, two drops of dilute 0.03% proparacaine solution can be instilled in the conjunctiva at 15 second intervals and 0.5% proparacaine instilled at 30 second intervals without pain. Four drops of 0.03% proparacaine and one minute intervals are required before a drop of 4% lidocaine is painless. Using 0.03% proparacaine, most patients will feel nothing except the cold of the solution. Eye drops can be made painless for children by this mechanism.

These dilute painless topical anesthetics should have extensive application in the emergency room and in environments where foreign objects and caustic substances can cause ocular injury. The dilute topical anesthetics do not induce squinting or squeezing of the lids—a decided advantage. The cornea can be irrigated with these solutions for pain-free removal of foreign material.

The dropper bottles of all the topical anesthetics can be contaminated by personnel touching the dropper bottle to eyelashes or lids and to the aspiration of particulate matter from the air. After squeezing to produce a drop, air enters the bottle to replace the volume. Syringes when used for this purpose are difficult to control.

The clinical strengths of local anesthetic solutions available commercially are listed in Table 2.1. Four percent lidocaine, despite the work of Marr,[42] has never been submitted by the manufacturer for FDA approval for ophthalmic use in the U.S., despite its lack of toxicity to the corneal epithelium. It is the mainstay ophthalmic topical anesthetic in Europe. Four percent lidocaine topical anesthetic is available for mucous membrane use in the United States, but the solution contains 4% methylparaben.

A formulation of 4% lidocaine for ophthalmic use should be available for U.S. clinicians. The pharmacist can transfer 4% lidocaine for cardiac use to sterile dropper bottles for ophthalmic use.

Physiology of Nerve Transmission

The nerve endings that transmit sharp pain are naked nerve endings in the skin, conjunctiva, and cornea. The skin nerve endings are covered with stratified cornified epithelium which is almost impermeable to local anesthetics; it is slightly permeable to benzocaine. A new eutectic mixture of lidocaine and prilocaine, called EMLA, has been introduced by Astra for application on the skin. It will produce anesthesia if contact with the skin is maintained for one hour. This preparation has been used successfully prior to retrobulbar blocks.[43]

The mucous membranes are covered by stratified epithelium which is not cornified and allows penetration of base local anesthetic. This is why the conjunctiva and the mucous membranes of the throat and GU tract can be topically anesthetized. Much anesthetic is lost in contact with body fluids and the epithelium, so high concentration and large volumes must be used. When this excess active drug is absorbed via the mucous membranes of the GI or GU tract or the lungs systemic toxicity becomes a problem.

The nerve endings in the cornea are superficial and extend between epithelial cells and are covered only by the tear film. Penetration into the corneal nerves requires transfer across the three layers of the tear film. The lipid layer will saturate rapidly with base form local anesthetic. Transfer across the aqueous layer requires cationic molecules. Transfer across the mucin layer is easier for the base form. Thus the tear film is a formidable challenge for molecular diffusion, but is facilitated by anesthetic in the pH range of 7.4 and molecules which have both lipid and aqueous solubility.

Instead of relying on pH and molecular design, most commercial preparations contain facilitators to chemically destroy the integrity of the tear film, such as benzalkonium chloride. The safety and efficacy of corneal topical anesthetics are very confusing because in laboratory experiments solutions were used which did not have such facilitators in them. The pH adjustment of local anesthetics into the range of tears (pH 7.8)

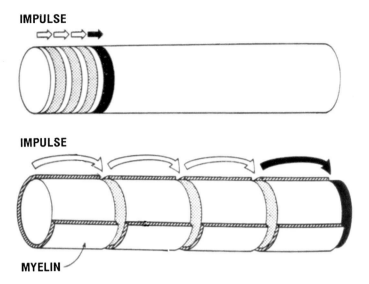

Figure 2.2. Above, a non-myelinated nerve is diagrammed. Spread of electrical impulse moves forward by sequentially depolarizing adjacent strips of nerve membrane on the periphery of the axon. The lower figure, a myelinated nerve, shows the myelin sheath partly stripped with the nodes of Ranvier seen as space between myelinated areas. Electrical impulse moves from one node to the next, but is able to jump over 2 or 3 nodes with no change or only partial block of axonal activity. A minimum of 3 to 5 nodes must be blocked with local anesthetic to produce failure of impulse propagation for that axon. (Courtesy R. de Jong, modified from his book *Local Anesthetics*).[49a]

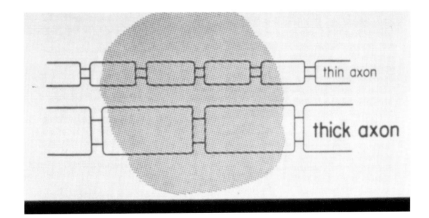

Figure 2.3. Myelinated nerves with thin axons are more readily blocked than large, thick axons. Motor nerves are more likely than sensory nerves to contain thick axons. (Courtesy R. de Jong, modified from his book *Local Anesthetics*).[49a]

Block of Sodium Channels

For local anesthetics to block nerve impulses, molecules must first diffuse into the nerve in adequate concentration. The diffusion of the drug from where it is deposited is a complex phenomenon because spread of local anesthetic occurs in all directions as does diffusion, so that the concentration of local anesthetic decreases rapidly as tissues chemically and physically bind anesthetic molecules. The local anesthetic then permeates the nerve to block the sodium channels (Figures 2.4-2.7).

There are millions of sodium channels per square millimeter of axon surface. The local anesthetics block the voltage-gated sodium channels preventing opening of the channels and inhibiting their activation.

Local anesthetics diffuse into the sodium channel and block sodium ions from entering the axons. When sodium channels are blocked, the nerve impulse is not propagated along an axon. However, it requires block of 3 to 7 mm of a myelinated nerve or 2 to 3 mm of a non-myelinated nerve to prevent propagation of the nerve impulse.

An incompletely blocked nerve will continue to conduct impulses, but at a lower

Figure 2.4. Local anesthetic is injected extraneurally to prevent nerve trauma. The concentration of blocking agent in the pool is diminished as it spreads toward the nerve sheath. The mantle fibers near the nerve's external surface are exposed first to the blocking agent. In this and the following figures, the anesthetic concentration is represented by density of shading, a white region representing a sub-C_m concentration, where C_m is the concentration of local anesthetic required in the axons to block axonal conduction in 10 minutes. Diffusion proceeds along the arrows down the concentration gradient. Only a single mantle and a core bundle are shown in the nerve. (Courtesy R. de Jong, modified from his book *Local Anesthetics*).[49a]

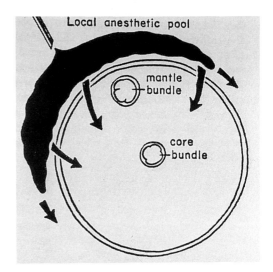

Figure 2.5. The anesthetic front has traversed the nerve's mantle region, bringing mantle fibers to C_m; impulse conduction through the mantle fibers has been halted. The diffusion front has not yet reached the core, so that conduction along core fibers continues uninterrupted. (Courtesy R. de Jong, modified from his book *Local Anesthetics*).[49a]

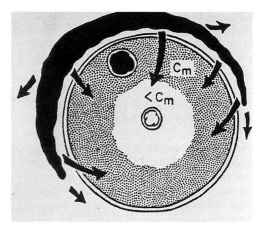

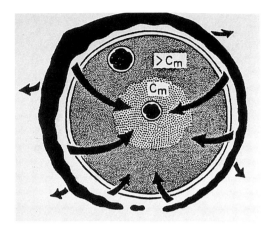

Figure 2.6. The anesthetic front, although weakened, reaches the core, bringing it to C_m. All fibers now are blocked and the innervated territory is anesthetized. Core fibers blocked later and exposed to a weaker anesthetic concentration, and thus may not be as solidly blocked as the mantle fibers. Because of a large pool of anesthetic, a mantle-to-core concentration gradient still exists; ultimately, the core's anesthetic content builds up well beyond C_m.

This would not be the case if anesthetic in minimal volume were placed in a tissue area of high absorption or rapid blood flow as in the orbit. In the orbit the core fibers may never reach C_m, even then the block might be partial if an inadequate length of nerve were blocked—see figure 2.10.(Courtesy R. de Jong, modified from his book *Local Anesthetics*).[49a]

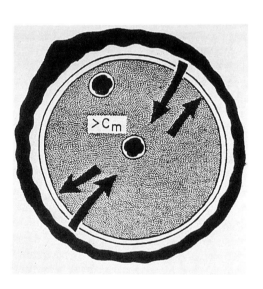

Figure 2.7. Diffusion, dispersion, dilution, absorption and binding continue. Ultimately, the intra- and extraneural concentrations equalize, and diffusion equilibrium is reached. (Courtesy R. de Jong, modified from his book *Local Anesthetics*).[49a]

frequency. As the anesthetic diffuses into a nerve it may block the outer axons but not the inner axons, causing a partial block (Figure 2.6). Stimulation of a sensory nerve with a partial block can be experienced as excruciating pain by some persons, whereas stimulation during total block is painless. Muscles partially blocked are weakened.

It is imperative that sufficient length of nerve be blocked as well as a sufficient depth of penetration of the nerve to have total blockade of the nerve (Figure 2.7).

Either or both can be the problem of total blockage of the motor fibers to the extraocular muscles; partial block is much more common from a single injection than total block. Furthermore, an incompletely blocked muscle is more likely to regain activity at a sooner time than one completely blocked. Augmentation from the same or a complementary injection site is often necessary for a total block that will not wear off prematurely.

Figure 2.8. With the extraneural drug reservoir depleted, the diffusion gradient reverses; local anesthetic begins to leave the nerve. (Courtesy R. de Jong, modified from his book *Local Anesthetics*).[49a]

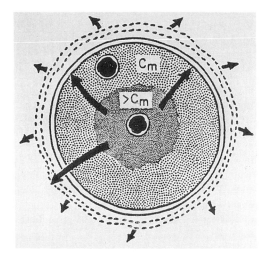

Figure 2.9. Mantle bundles lose local anesthetic faster than core bundles. Core fibers may remain blocked after the mantle's anesthetic concentration has dropped below C_m. The sensory areas of muscles first blocked recover function, while that blocked last remains anesthetized. The block begins to regress, but differently than it was blocked. (Courtesy R. de Jong, modified from his book *Local Anesthetics*).[49a]

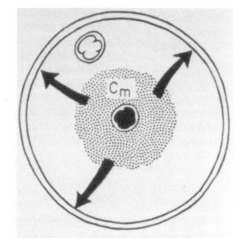

During onset and recovery from local anesthesia impulse blockade is incomplete, and partially blocked fibers are further inhibited by repetitive stimulation that produces an additional use-dependent binding to sodium channels (Figures 2.5, 2.8, 2.9).

The rates of onset and recovery from blockade are covered by relatively slow diffusion of local anesthetic molecules into and out of the nerve, and not by the rate at which the molecules bind and dissociate into the sodium ion channels.

Pharmacodynamics of Clinically Useful Local Anesthetics

The clinically important properties of the local anesthetics include potency, speed of onset, duration of anesthetic action, and differential sensory/motor blockade. These qualities vary from one drug to another.

Potency is primarily related to the lipophilic action of the molecule since it must penetrate the lipid layer of nerve membranes. This characteristic causes penetration of all cells, not just nerves—the more lipophilic, the more potent and the more toxic to cardiac cells.

The potency of local anesthetics, though related to their lipophilic chemical nature, is also a strict chemical configuration phenomenon intrinsic to the molecule.

Potency varies with the amount of vasodilatation, which causes the local anesthetic to be removed before it actually penetrates the nerve. Furthermore, the more lipid soluble anesthetics are, the more likely that they will be taken up by other tissues. The very rapidly perfused orbital connective tissue is, thus, a significant barrier to diffusion of local anesthetics and the primary reason why local anesthetics injected in one area of the orbit do not necessarily diffuse in anesthetic concentration over significant distances. Orbits of patients with obese faces, the collagen-filled orbits of patients with Graves' disease, and the fluid-filled orbits of prednisone users contain extra tissues to absorb anesthetic.

Bergen has shown that the orbital adipose tissue compartments have an extensive micro-circulation.[47] Arteries move from posterior to anterior, and the veins run from anterior to posterior. Thus a counter-current flow extraction process is possible (Figure 2.10-2.11).

The orbit has not been studied by radio-isotopic local anesthetic molecules, only by studying radio-opaque substances added to solutions. Because of the difference in

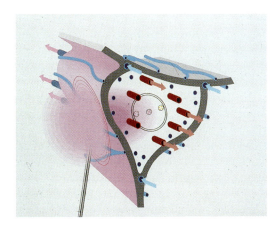

Figure 2.10. Blocking the oculomotor nerve with 4 ml of 4% lidocaine or 0.75% bupivacaine from a single site, despite an orbital volume of 30 ml often leads to a partial block, which clinically regresses more rapidly than when akinesia is produced. The connective tissue septa, the vascular adipose tissue compartments (ATC's), and the varying depth of the orbit combine to produce both effects.

When the anesthetic is injected into a pool at the anterior end of a ATC or in an adjacent ATC, there is rapid loss of concentration as the pool approaches the nerve. That diminished pool concentration reduces rapidly because of the counter current blood flow in the orbit.

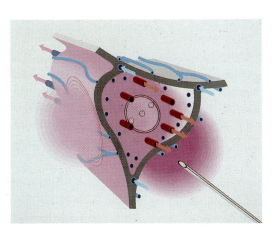

Figure 2.11. When akinesia is desired or a long-lasting block is sought, it makes good sense to plan a supplemental injection before the anesthetic concentration in the original pool is exhausted. Supplementation from an adjacent site rather than adding to the original pool can be highly efficacious.

properties of these materials, the distribution of radio-opaque solution and the distribution of anesthetic molecules may be orders of magnitude in difference.

The onset of action of local anesthetics is partly related to their physicochemical properties, to the concentration of the local anesthetic injection and to the pH of the solution. Onset is related to the number of base form molecules present in the area surrounding the nerve or lipid layers of tear film which is a function of the pK_a and the pH of the surrounding medium.

As the pH of the anesthetic solution or of the surrounding medium is increased, more molecules of local anesthetic are present in the base form, which should increase diffusion of anesthetics of base form into the nerve, provided the saturation point for precipitation of base form does not occur. However, in an area of rapid blood flow like the orbital connective tissue, transcapillary extraction is also facilitated as concentration of base form predominates. pH adjustment of the local anesthetics bottled at pH of 6 or above to reach 7.4 has minimal effect, and pH adjustment of local anesthetic bupivacaine solutions, although reported to greatly facilitate onset of local anesthetic activity by Zahl,[31] has failed to make a significant contribution in the hands of the authors.

On the other hand, solutions of local anesthetic with epinephrine are bottled at pH of 3 to 3.5 and pH adjustment is probably effective in facilitating onset, as well as decreasing pain. The authors discourage the use of these premixed anesthetic solutions with epinephrine in the orbit because of their high concentration of metabisulfite, since this substance is allergenic and neurotoxic.

The authors recommend the addition of 0.1 ml of 1:1000 epinephrine at time of use to 20 ml ampules or vials, or 0.15 ml of 1:1000 to 30 ml vials, to produce 1:200,000 solutions. One of the authors adds epinephrine in this concentration to mepivacaine, the other author adds the equivalent of 0.08 ml to mepivacaine solutions to give a concentration between 1:250,000 and 1:300,000. The use of this amount of epinephrine as a marker of inadvertent intravenous injection is encouraged. It facilitates augmentation and longer action of lidocaine, mepivacaine, bupivacaine, or etidocaine.

Rate of onset of motor block is complex in the orbit and varies with volume, time, concentration, and site of injection. de Jong defines minimal local anesthetic concentration as that concentration which will produce clinical block in 10 minutes.[48,49] The authors define a 50% akinesia as that time when, if muscle is blocked less than 50%, it will probably never be completely blocked. Noting this time allows one to plan supplemental or augmentation in a realistic fashion.

The 50% akinesia time corresponds to four minutes with 2% mepivacaine with 1:200,000 epinephrine and hyaluronidase and five minutes for a mixture of one part 2% mepivacaine with two parts 0.75% bupivacaine with 1:250,000 epinephrine and 0.75 iu hyaluronidase per milliliter. Clinically, if akinesia has not reached 50% at the 50% akinesia time, one should plan on augmenting the block, if 100% akinesia is desired. Both the authors provide virtually all their patients for intraocular surgery with total akinesia. Knowing when to augment is clinically important.

Augmentation should not be done in less than five minutes because it is unwise to place more anesthetic in the orbit than the orbit will tolerate and cannot be done without raising the intraocular pressure above 25 to 30 mmHg. Most orbits will decompress adequately in five to seven minutes for augmentation of a volume similar to that of the preceding injection if orbital massage is started immediately after the injection is complete. That is to say, if the initial injection was limited to 4 ml because orbital pressure rose, then with orbital decompression of five to seven minutes, an additional

4 ml of anesthetic can probably be placed in the orbit. Pressure rise is often less. It is important, however, to observe the rate of progression of orbital pressure as the secondary filling occurs. As discussed in Chapter One, orbits vary greatly in their sensitivity to increasing pressure with increasing injections.

Using this philosophy, both authors have provided 100% akinesia for the last 5,000 cases each has performed. Complete akinesia for the patient, in addition to eliminating tension of the muscles on the globe, provides complete anesthesia since most motor nerves require two to four times the concentration for total block that sensory and sympathetic nerves do. However, if akinesia occurs with a 2 ml injection of local anesthetic at the bifurcation of the oculomotor nerve deep in the apex, then it is likely that the ciliary ganglion will be blocked, but it is unlikely that anesthesia of the infraorbital nerve will occur. Injections in the mid-orbit can provide total akinesia and anesthesia when adequate volume is injected.

The duration of action of local anesthetics is related to their chemical characteristics and to the amount of blood flow in the area surrounding the nerve. Most local anesthetics have a bi-phasic action. Most local anesthetics in very low concentration cause vasoconstriction, and at a slightly higher concentration, cause vasodilatation.[50] The vasodilatation then causes more rapid extraction of the drug away from the site. Lidocaine is a more potent vasodilator than mepivacaine. It is thought that this may be related to the shorter duration of activity of lidocaine. In the orbit 1:200,000 epinephrine provides significant prolongation of mepivacaine and lidocaine block in the authors' experience.

Mepivacaine reputedly has a vasoconstrictive activity much greater than that of lidocaine or bupivacaine, which led to its introduction into dentistry as the agent which would cause vasoconstriction and not require additional epinephrine.

Duration of action of all local anesthetics, in the final analysis, is more related to hydrophobicity than to lipophilicity and to the intrinsic chemical nature of the agent itself than to any other factors.

The differential effect of local anesthetics on sensory and motor nerves has been alluded to previously. This phenomenon was not recognized until the development of etidocaine. Etidocaine diffuses into a mixed nerve, rapidly blocking it, but diffuses out of the sensory nerves leaving a prolonged block of the motor nerve and no sensory anesthesia. In general surgery this caused many patients great anxiety and led to a limited use of the drug. However, in ophthalmology, for procedures in which prolonged akinesia is desirable, the drug could have considerable use.

On the other hand, bupivacaine tends to diffuse into nerves much more slowly—to solidly block the sensory nerves and more slowly block motor nerves. It then usually diffuses out the motor nerves prior to or at the same time it leaves the sensory nerves. In the orbit there is often a long motor block with the higher 0.75% bupivacaine. Therefore, these two drugs can be used differentially in ophthalmology in cases where prolonged akinesia is thought to be in the patient's best interest. The high cost and pain of injection with etidocaine have limited its usefulness, however.

Efficacy studies of local anesthetics in ophthalmology are few. Swan did his classical work on the subconjunctival administration of procaine as causing transfer of local anesthetic into the aqueous, iris, and choroid. The authors are unaware of any comparable studies showing the clinical effectiveness of other drugs. For instance, did cocaine 4% mixed equally with 1:1,000 epinephrine actually produce clinical block of pain fibers in the iris, as noted by O'Brien[51] or was it a clinical circumstance that patients did not complain of pain?

Obviously the closer to the nerve an injection is placed, the more rapid the onset and the lower the concentration of the injected drug that is requried. The closer to the nerve, however, the more risk of damage to it or to the associated arteries and veins. The higher the concentration of drug, the higher the concentration in arteries or veins if they are inadvertently injected. Therefore, rapid onset, effectiveness, and safety can be mutually exclusive.

However, if local anesthetics are injected very slowly, and the needle moved to ensure it is not within a blood vessel, then rapid onset and effectiveness can be accomplished safely, and the greater the distance from the nerve, the greater the safety because in most areas of the body the nerve, artery, and vein are close.

This close relationship of vein, artery, and nerve is not true in the orbit, where arteries and veins often do not run together. The larger veins usually run in the septa, and the venules empty into them. The arteries merely pierce the septa before subdividing to provide profuse micro-circulation of the adipose tissue compartments.[47]

All local anesthetic drugs tend to show a process called augmentation.[50b] If a local anesthetic is injected into an area and incomplete blockade ensues, it is possible to inject the same area with a similar or smaller dosage of local anesthetic of the same concentration and following injection of that second dose, the block will become much more profound. Total block of nerves can be elicited by this technique. Augmentation also tends to promote a longer lasting block, especially if the nerve block is augmented about the time the local anesthetic would be expected to wear off (Figure 2.11).

Augmentation has clinical usefulness in ophthalmic anesthesia if one dose of local anesthetic does not tend to produce akinesia. It is then possible to inject into the same or an adjacent area and add local anesthetic. In the orbit, however, with its rapid blood flow, augmentation may not be effective if the duration between primary and secondary injection is too great—the authors feel that augmentation is present for 20 minutes but have not studied longer time intervals.

Choosing the Optimal Local Anesthetic Drug

Table 2.1 contains the clinically useful concentrations of the local anesthetics and their intended use, as well as their trade names.

Lidocaine has the fastest onset, but the shortest duration. Three ml of a 1% concentration placed 5 to 7 mm behind the hind surface of the globe at the opening of the muscle cone will usually provide dilatation of the pupil indicating block of the ciliary ganglion and/or ciliary nerves within 10 or 15 seconds. Onset of corneal anesthesia occurs within a minute, and a minor effect on motor activity of the extraocular muscles in 90% of patients, but a significant motor block in 10%; 1% lidocaine will last from 20 minutes to an hour.

Two percent lidocaine will block the ciliary ganglion in approximately the same period of time and provide complete block of the extraocular muscles in five to 10 minutes in 75% of patients and will last for 45 minutes to two hours; 4% lidocaine will produce complete akinesia in five minutes in 75%, and in 90% by 10 minutes, but produce little or no akinesia in the remaining 10% of patients and will last from one to three hours. Augmentation is effective with lidocaine.

Duration is quite variable with lidocaine. It is not uncommon for 4% to wear off in 30 to 45 minutes in persons with high levels of anxiety; this effect is probably due to blood flow or some other phenomenon, as yet incompletely understood in anxious people.

Local anesthetics tend to wear off much more rapidly in people who use excessive alcohol, nicotine, and barbiturates, in the opinion of the authors. These persons are much more likely to benefit from augmentation of their block if adequate duration of anesthesia is required or if post-operative analgesia is desired. If foreknowledge is available, bupivacaine 0.75% with epinephrine is the drug of choice. Epinephrine is essential to adequate blocks in such people, and augmentation is often necessary.

Nifedipine therapy is often associated with rapid drug washout unless epinephrine is used. Interestingly, a suspected side-effect of this medication is the symptom of facial flushing. This flushing is common with beta-blocker therapy.

Mepivacaine of the same concentration as lidocaine has a slightly slower onset of activity, but in the orbit, will usually last one and a half to two times as long as lidocaine when injected in the same strength and with the same amount of epinephrine.

Bupivacaine has an onset very much related to concentration; 0.25% is very slow and will often produce little akinesia; whereas, 0.75% is very similar to 2% mepivacaine in onset. Duration is also very sensitive to concentration and to the use of epinephrine. 0.75% bupivacaine will last from 2.5 to 24 hours. Refer to Table 2.1 for the estimated clinical times.

Etidocaine is also concentration dependent. The 0.5% is similar to 1% lidocaine; 1% is much like 2-4% lidocaine.

The authors are convinced that epinephrine extends the analgesia and akinesia time of lidocaine and mepivacaine, and one author believes the same is true for bupivacaine. Extended analgesia time provides much more pleasant post-operative course.

Systemic Toxicity

The amide local anesthetics tend to produce a recognizable symptom/complex related to the venous blood concentration, even though this concentration measured in peripheral venous blood may be deceivingly lower than the heart and brain effect because of considerable first pass extraction of anesthetic in the lung. Therefore, measured peripheral intravenous concentrations do not necessarily relate to the actual arterial concentration in the coronary arteries. The mixing in the venous blood en route to the lungs and heart effects the mean concentration significantly.

The first sign or symptom of systemic toxicity is usually circum-oral or tongue numbness, then lightheadedness or tinnitus, followed by visual disturbances, muscular twitching, then convulsions and unconsciousness. Respiratory arrest occurs at almost twice the concentration required to produce unconsciousness. Lidocaine and mepivacaine, at levels producing respiratory arrest, usually produce some decrease in cardiac output, and the EKG remains relatively stable with some increase in P-R interval and QRS duration.

Bupivacaine has profoundly adverse effects on conduction in the heart, where the molecule actually enters cardiac cells and only slowly exits. High concentration can lead to torsades de Pointes in which resuscitation is very difficult.[52,53] Bupivacaine should always be injected very slowly and with epinephrine as a marker to signal intravenous injection. This phenomenon of epinephrine causing slight tachycardia immediately after injection is more reliable in the orbit than in the epidural space; the epinephrine will help to reduce the adverse effect of the bupivacaine.

Profound CNS effects can occur with rapid injection of local anesthetic into the head or neck because of retrograde flow into the brain from either arteries or veins. This bizarre, potentially lethal complication can only be prevented by slow injection.

The convulsive activity of local anesthetics is thought to be related to blockade of inhibitors in the brainstem, not by causing a hyperexcitable effect on the motor cortex. Early in the history of local anesthetic toxicity studies, it was thought that the barbiturates would prevent convulsions and were specifically beneficial at preventing CNS toxicity; however, recent studies have failed to confirm this.[49c] The amide local anesthetics are fair anticonvulsants.[49b] The benzodiazepines appear to have significant benefit in prevention and treatment of local anesthetic seizure.[49c]

Prevention and Management of Systemic Toxicity

Prevention of local anesthetic toxicity is a matter of minimizing blood concentration. Reducing blood concentration can be accomplished by slow injection, slow pick-up of anesthetic from the tissue in which it has been deposited, and avoiding intravascular injection of the local anesthetic drug. Rarely does orbital block approach 75% of the accepted maximum safe dose of local anesthetic; however, the higher concentration of local anesthetics, e.g., 0.75% bupivacaine and 4% lidocaine, do add up rapidly. Prudence and accurate reading of labels are essential to safety.

Local anesthetic injections in the head and neck area are riskier because of retrograde spread of local anesthetic if injected at a high rate either in an artery or a vein. High injection rate in an orbital vein can cause retrograde flow back into the brain with onset of convulsions, even though the concentration measured in the venous blood may be inconsequential. The actual concentration in the brain will be the important determinant.

High injection rate into a branch of the facial or internal carotid artery can cause retrograde flow into the brain with much greater brain effect than would be seen from the same amount of local anesthetic injected intravenously. Thus slow injection in the orbit is mandatory. There is no reason to exceed the pain producing rate of 1 ml in any 10 second interval.

Local anesthetic injected in the sheath of the optic nerve can move subdurally or in the subarachnoid space along the optic chiasm into the subarachnoid space of the other eye or into the midbrain causing apnea, sympathetic blockade, or vagal blockade with varying cardiovascular effects (see Chapter 4). Brainstem anesthesia is thus induced. However, that is not the only route by which brainstem anesthesia can happen. Transfer across the intact dura, and hydraulic dissection along the dural cleavage zone of the attachment of the dura to the skull at the orbital apex are other mechanisms. Zahl has reported the latter for peribulbar anesthesia.[54]

The Useful Role of Sedatives in Local Anesthesia

Since the early clinical introduction of barbiturates into ophthalmic and anesthesia practice, the relationship of pre-operative sedation to the success of local anesthetic technique has been controversial. In the hands of some physicians and anesthesia providers, sedatives have been a tremendous boon, for other people they have caused loss of vision and death.

The early writers recognized that these drugs often provided a calm and tranquil patient; on the other hand, many persons seemed to become even more anxious after receiving them for sedation. For that reason, Atkinson encouraged the hospitalization of patients so they could receive their first dose of sedative the night before surgery to determine its efficacy. The administration of a subsequent dose of sedative in the morning before surgery and more drugs when patients arrived in the operating room was recommended.

The authors believe that the most important sedative a patient can have is the knowledge that the operation on an eye, such as cataract surgery, is more anxiety producing for most patients than any other operation they will have for the rest of their lives. The vast majority of patients who have any emotional or cardiovascular stress from anxiety will demonstrate this the night before or the morning of cataract surgery. The knowledge that this is a normal response is very helpful. We do not believe that mild doses of sedatives changes this stress response picture, in fact, we believe that in some cases, it is made worse.

Those persons who react with hypertension and tachycardia need drugs specific for these responses, either by referral to their local physician for ongoing medical therapy for systemic hypertension, carcinoid states, hyperthyroidism, etc. or treatment the day of cataract surgery by the anesthesia provider.

Sub-lingual nifedipine, in both authors' practices, is quite beneficial as the first step for systolic pressure above 170 mmHg. If the systolic hypertension continues after nifedipine, one of the authors administers hydralazine and/or propranolol in small, divided doses of 0.25 mg propranolol or 5 mg hydralazine to control the systemic hypertension before injecting around and behind the eye and to provide reasonable systolic pressure during surgery. A painless block can then be done without inducing further cardiovascular stress or increasing the risk of bleeding if the patient is cooperative.

If the patient is anxious or systolic hypertension persists, then a dose of 25 to 75 mg thiopental and/or midazolam 0.3 mg will usually cause enough venous dilatation to get blood pressure below 155 mmHg during the block and keep it there to provide good intra-operative control. Propofol® may become the sedative of choice for such anxious hypertensives.

If the patient is really anxious, but not hypertensive, then a small dose of thiopental (37.5 mg) or midazolam (0.3 mg) or both or propotol 15 mg can be very beneficial and analgesic.[62]

Certain patients are extremely anxious about having injections around the eye and are extremely squinty; as Wright so aptly described, their whole face will "screw up."[55] This special group of patients can be approached by doing a Nadbath, O'Brien, or Atkinson block of the facial nerve first, but the authors prefer to use 5 mg of oral diazepam 30 minutes before the block and/or midazolam 0.3 mg intravenously; if the patient then becomes totally cooperative, the block is performed in the usual manner. If the patient is not totally cooperative and cannot refrain from blinking, then the authors make the primary injection through the medial canthus or through an area in the inferior lid just at the edge of the tarsal plate at the lateral canthus. These areas do not move when people squint, and using painless technique, it is possible to place the needle correctly and start anesthetization of the orbit and pre-septal branches of the facial nerve to the orbicularis muscle.

Brevital®, Pentothal®, and midazolam alone or accompanied by a narcotic are commonly administered to induce a temporary short state of anesthesia which allows the injections around and behind the eye to be done without the patient being aware of the injections. One of the authors used this technique on some 10,000 consecutive patients and found it was very reliable in the hands of two anesthesia trained personnel—one to administer the drug and maintain the airway, and the other to make the injections of local anesthetic.

The disadvantages of the technique are twofold: (1) Those persons who are the most frightened usually require a far greater dose of the drug than does the average person to prevent them from suddenly squinting, coughing, or pulling away from the anesthetist, and if the injections exceed the pain threshold, the patient may cause self injury. (2) The patient will be unable to signal proximity of the needle to structures in the orbit which will elicit pain with needle touch and allow the needle to be withdrawn prior to damage to the structure.

When an anesthetic state (unconscious sedation) is induced for the block, it is mandatory that the person making the injection have a deep understanding of orbital anatomy and geometry because structures can be contacted with the needle and damaged with no feedback from the patient.

When this brief anesthetic state is induced to make the block painless, it is wise to stimulate the patient first in some area besides the orbit to ascertain the lack of responsiveness of the patient to painful stimuli; otherwise, if the pain threshold is exceeded by a needle in the orbit, the patient may suddenly move in a more uncontrollable manner than they would if awake. Perforation of the globe, optic nerve, or ophthalmic artery can ensue.

If one uses the short general anesthesia method to truly produce absence of painful response and can establish the state exists, then the injections can be placed in the orbit with more safety for that patient than they would be if the patient were awake and over-reacting or sedated but not in control, providing the blocker has the requisite skill and mechanical dexterity to by-pass the patient's pain defenses. This less than optimal state can be chosen by patient and provider with informed consent for these patients unable to control themselves.

By reducing injection rate of local anesthetic and making preliminary injections of painless local anesthetic, the need for unconscious sedation in 99.5% of patients can be eliminated. One hundred percent of these patients will be happy with the painless nature of their eye block.

The authors believe strongly that sedatives should not be used to abolish the pain in the back, neck, or extremities caused by arthritis and bad pre-operative positioning. The art of primary care—supporting heads, necks, and extremities—is extremely important to safe local anesthesia management. This must be primary.

The elderly can be placed in dangerous positions that compromise basilar artery flow if the neck is hyper-extended. Sedation in such a position can cause death by brain stem infarction.

The authors believe that sedatives should not be used to treat the patient who responds to a painful stimulus when the patient complains that the operation is hurting them under local anesthesia. The treatment of choice is to inject local anesthetic into the innervation of the area before proceeding with surgery under all except the most emergent conditions.

One such emergency occurs when a patient starts to have vitreous prolapse or expulsive hemorrhage. It is reported that such patients will feel pain, even though prior to the onset of the episode, they were considered to have a perfect block and be pain-free. The authors doubt that the patient truly had a total block to begin with, and consider that patient most likely had an incomplete block which had not been adequately tested prior to surgery or an early fading of the block.

Neither author has found that choroidal effusion has been painful in a totally blocked eye, in the approximately six cases in which they have seen it in their combined 36,000 cases. Only one author has seen a single expulsive hemorrhage, and it was painless.

If the patient is beginning to move and there is iris prolapse or signs of choroidal effusion and a tight globe, the patient must be temporarily constrained to prevent them from holding their breath or coughing or bucking. This is a sight-saving emergency. Intravenous general anesthesia is warranted to provide adequate operating conditions, and immediate intravenous mannitol. For this reason, the authors have Pentothal or Brevital drawn up and mannitol warmed to body temperature in the operating room at all times to handle that emergency. The new drug, propofol, may be more beneficial in this circumstance, but the authors have no experience with it. Local pain in the vein caused by the drug could make matters worse.

The authors are convinced that people who have an incomplete block are more likely to have choroidal effusion or expulsive hemorrhage and that the sympathetic activity induced by inadequate anesthetization of the orbit may well be one of the primary factors in this process.

Expulsive hemorrhage occurred under general anesthesia in the classical video of Girard during bucking on an endotracheal tube. The authors wonder if the course of events was not lightening of anesthesia from "pain" of choroidal or iris origin followed by sympathetic visceral pain with abnormal choroidal blood flow inducing the choroidal effusion. That "pain" was "antidote" to the level of "anesthesia" and the resulting inadequate level of anesthesia induced bucking. The actual bucking on the tube, though deleterious from a venous return point of view and aggravating the effusion, may well have been secondary to the cause of the episode.

The authors believe that intravenous mannitol is the primary drug for the treatment of choroidal effusion or iris prolapse and have this drug warmed to body temperature and available in the operating room for immediate treatment. Bolus mannitol lowers vitreous volume in three minutes.

The Harmful Role of Sedatives in Local Anesthesia for Ophthalmic Procedures

Sedatives make it difficult to determine whether the eye is totally anesthetized. One cannot establish ocular akinesia in the very drugged person because of their inability to move the control eye through 100% of arc, even if they transiently arouse to attempt it.

Sedatives also allow persons to lie in uncomfortable positions and then emerge from that position at an unexpected time; this is especially true with cervical stenosis and basilar artery insufficiency which can lead to disorientation and fighting for life. This type of activity or moving because of pain can lead to contamination of the wound or expulsive hemorrhage.

For these reasons, we believe that sedatives should not have a primary role in ophthalmic local anesthesia, except for the rare patient who is uncooperative for a block. Such patients occasionally require further consideration in the operating room due to their fear or inability to cooperate. Such patients are best handled in the operating room with light general anesthesia rather than just heavy sedation, after they have a perfect augmented block.

The authors choose a local anesthetic that outlasts the longest operation. For surgery longer than two hours, the authors prefer total local anesthetic block, supplemented by light general anesthesia and augmentation of the local anesthetic by the surgeon during and at the end of the operation.

Allergy to Local Anesthetics

The treatment of acute allergic response is a major emergency. It is fortunate that allergy to the amide local anesthetics is an extremely rare event. The authors, in their combined practices of more than 36,000 cases, have never seen an acute allergy to the amide local anesthetics or to hyaluronidase.

The allergic potential of the ester local anesthetics and the fact that amide local anesthetics can do the same job has been discussed. The only ester local anesthetic that the authors believe has any place is proparacaine, and that drug does not break down into para-aminobenzoic acid, the high allergen. Inserting dilute proparacaine, telling the patient one is injecting a test dose, and allowing time to show any acute ocular manifestations is psychologically beneficial to any patient with great concern about allergy.

Likewise, one author makes a test injection of the local anesthetic to be used for the eye block in the skin on the dorsum of the arm or the hand, and a test dose in the conjunctival area prior to injection of the full-strength local anesthetic drug. The injection is done to relieve the pain of starting an IV and the pain of making the first injection of local anesthetic. However, it is beneficial to review the test dose areas before the block and one to two hours later or the next day and establish that there are no signs of unusual wheal formation.

If the ester local anesthetics are used, we believe a test injection is necessary in the skin to exclude allergy to those drugs. In this we agree with Aldrete.[56]

Allergy to hyaluronidase has been reported, but the report occurred many years ago when the process of purification was not at its current level. Nonetheless, a test dose of the local anesthetic containing hyaluronidase in the skin is routine for one of the authors. The site of the test injection is noted and minutes or hours later can be examined for signs of skin allergy.

Neurotoxicity and Myotoxicity

In the early days of conduction anesthesia, injection directly into a nerve trunk was considered innocuous and totally reversible. Injection into muscles was also considered innocuous. Today we know that injection into these structures is not innocuous (see Chapter 4—myotoxicity). There are reports of irreversible damage to peripheral nerves in which the symptom of acute paresthesia was elicited at time of the injection; the injection could have been intraneural or the vascular integrity of the nerve compromised.

Today nerve block techniques rely upon eliciting a paresthesia with an electrical stimulus rather than with the needle itself, or to administering local anesthetics into a compartment or area where there is no need of paresthesia to locate the point of the needle.

The orbit, because of the five adipose tissue compartments, allows an almost perfect situation for this skill of "compartment anesthesia" to be performed. It is not necessary to place a needle close to the optic, oculomotor, abducens, or trochlear nerves, nor into any of the foramina to block the supraorbital nerve, zygomaticofacial nerve, or the infraorbital nerves. Blocks of these two latter nerves can be done outside the orbit in the preseptal space by using bulk spread technique.

Therefore, we would like to think that the problem of neurotoxicity in the orbit is totally eliminated. However, reports of blindness following injection of local anesthetic still occur. Whether these are injections into the nerve itself or damage to its blood supply is unknown. Injection of local anesthetic directly into the globe has been reported with lidocaine with the patient recovering to 20/20 vision.[56] The authors of that report describe reduction of intraocular pressure by paracentesis, but questioned whether it was, in fact, vision-saving.

There is no question that the local anesthetic drugs are myotoxic. When injected within the sheath of any muscle so far studied, the local anesthetics above a threshold concentration cause myonecrosis with loss of myotubules. The damaged fibers become hyalinized and there is an invasion of the fibers by macrophages. However, the cell nuclei seem to be spared. Regeneration starts after several days and is complete in four to six weeks if the micro-circulation of the nerve and muscle are intact.

Myonecrosis has been described with all local anesthetics and does not seem to be related to ester or amide linkage. The myotoxic effect of the local anesthetic is concentration dependent, dependent upon the volume of muscle into which it is injected, and to the presence of limited epimysial or perimysial spread. Thus the extraocular muscles should be good candidates for myonecrosis from intramuscular injection. Since damage is much more likely to be irreversible if the blood supply to the muscle is damaged, injection into the extraocular muscles in the area of the hilum should be scrupulously avoided.

The local anesthetics display some specificity with respect to myotoxic damage. Lidocaine preferentially destroys white fibers, whereas bupivacaine is more toxic to red fibers. However, at higher concentrations the specificity is lost and all striated muscle is damaged. Other tissues like connective tissue, neurons, and smooth muscle remain unaffected at the same concentration of local anesthetic.

Several authors have described clinical courses compatible with myotoxicity in which regeneration,[58,59,60] or restoration of normal function, occurred after two weeks to three months with no residual effects. On the other hand, other authors have described permanent residual diplopia.[61] Whether the latter is due to nerve supply damage of the muscle or to the onset of fibrosis is not clearly defined. However, either is a likely possibility.

Early recognition of myotoxicity and selective patching of the eye during regeneration is essential.

The Ideal Local Anesthetic

The criteria for an ideal local anesthetic would be:
- non-irritating
- non-pain producing
- no neurotoxicity
- no toxicity to any of the peripheral organs of the body, and
- dissolvable in a sterile and stable solution.

In this regard, the present amide local anesthetics come close in ophthalmology because of the smaller amounts of local anesthetic required to render the operative field pain-free and immobile. In other branches of surgery, it would be optimal to have local anesthetics that were more rapidly broken down by the body so that a larger total dosage could be administered without causing cardiovascular or central nervous system effects. No clinically useful commercial concentrations of local anesthetics have been found that produce painless injection. Therefore, the use of a painless dilute solution of local anesthetic is required for the provider wishing to anesthetize the patient without producing pain; pH adjustment and slow injection alleviate much pain.

Clinical Conclusion

Pharmacology of the amide local anesthetics has been studied sufficiently and drugs currently used allow the conjunctiva, the cornea, or the whole orbit to be anesthetized safely and without pain. Since the injection of local anesthetics in the bulbar conjunctiva and in the space between Tenon's and the sclera requires an extreme degree of skill to prevent injury, this route of administration of anesthetics is not recommended except for those few skilled surgeon/anesthetists or anesthesia providers who can accomplish it.

On the other hand, injections of local anesthetic in the mid-orbit can anesthetize the entire globe and all the extraocular muscles if sufficient volume is placed there in a reasonable volume single injection or by augmentation. The drug flows anteriorly or can be purposefully injected in the pre-septal space of the lid to block the orbicularis muscle and sensory nerves to the lids and conjunctiva. Thus we can provide total anesthesia, analgesia, and akinesia for all surgical procedures in the orbit.

The amide local anesthetics vary in onset time, duration of block, and their selectivity for sensory or motor nerves. The process of block augmentation is very germane to orbital anesthesia because often a single injection in one area will provide incomplete anesthesia or akinesia. Therefore, the anesthesia provider should know those areas to make such supplemental injections.

The danger of injecting local anesthetics intravenously or intra-arterially in the orbit in high concentration or at a high rate of injection is stressed because of the risk of retrograde flow into the brain and because of the risk of cardiac toxicity out of proportion to the amount of drug injected.

The risk of brain stem anesthesia can be reduced to almost zero by placing needles in the mid-orbit and using reasonable volumes of anesthetic and augmentation.

Local anesthetics can be prepared which are painless topically and by infiltration. A method of doing this has been described until an ideal local anesthetic is discovered.

Anesthetization with local anesthetics is an art as well as a science, and only when the technical aspects of administration are closely controlled and the provider's capability thoroughly assessed will the patient have maximum safety. Technique and technical skill will be considered in the next chapter.

References

1. Knapp H. On cocaine and its use in ophthalmic and general surgery. Arch Ophthalmol 13:402;1884.
2. Duverger. L'anesthésie locale en ophtalmologie. Masson et Cie, Paris, 1920.
3. Lowenstein A. Ueber regionare anasthesie in der orbita. Klin Monatsb f Augenh 592-601;1908.
4. Koller C(K). The use of local anesthesia on the eye. Preliminary report. Translation of Koller's preliminary report of Sept 15, 1884. Presented by Dr. Brettaur in: (eds) Faulconer A, Keys TE. Foundations of Anesthesiology. Charles C. Thomas, Springfield, 1965.
5. Koller K. On the use of cocaine to anaesthetize the eye. As translated by H Knapp in On Cocaine and Its Use in Ophthalmic and General Surgery. Arch Ophthalmol 13:402-48;1884. Translation of Koller's early pharmacology as reported in Oct 25 and Nov 1, Wein Med Wochenscreib 1884.
6. Braun H. Local Anesthesia. Translated and edited by Harris ML. Loa & Febiger, Philadelphia, 1924. p 239.
7. Pitkin GP. Conduction Anesthesia. Ed. Southworth JL, Hingson RA. JB Lippincott Co., Philadelphia, 1946. p 337. Second Edition, 1953, p 410.
8. O'Brien CS. Local anesthesia. Arch Ophthalmol 12:241-53;1934.
9. Atkinson WS. Local anesthesia in ophthalmology. Tr Am Ophth Soc 32:399-451;1934.
10. Atkinson WS. Local anesthesia in ophthalmology. Am J Ophthalmol 31:1607-18;1948.
11. Atkinson WS. Anesthesia in Ophthalmology, First Edition. Charles C. Thomas, Springfield, 1955.
12. Atkinson WS. Larger volume retrobulbar injections. Am J Ophthalmol 57:328;1964.
13. Atkinson WS. Anesthesia in Ophthalmology, Second Edition. Charles C. Thomas, Springfield, 1965.
14. Russell DA, Guyton JS. Retrobulbar injection of lidocaine (Xylocaine) for anesthesia and akinesia. Am J Ophthalmol 38:78-84;1954.
15. Wightman MA, Vaughan RW. Comparison of compounds used for intradermal anesthesia. Anesthesiology 45:687-9;1976.
16. Kirsch RE. Further studies on the use of digital pressure in cataract surgery. Arch Ophthalmol 58:641-4;1957.
17. Scheie HG, Ellis RA, et al. Long-lasting local anesthetic agents in ophthalmic surgery. Arch Ophthalmol 53:177-90;1955.
18. Laaka V, Nikki P, Tarkkanen A. Comparison of bupivacaine with and without adrenalin and mepivacaine with adrenalin in intraocular surgery. Acta Ophthalmol 50:229-39;1972.
19. Gills JP, Rudisill JE. Bupivacaine in cataract surgery. Ophthalmic Surg 5:67-70;1974.
20. Gutman H, Sinskey RM, et al. A comparison of lidocaine and etidocaine in retrobulbar anesthesia for cataract surgery. Am Intra-ocular Implant Soc J 5:120-22;1979.
21. Miller RD (ed). Anesthesia, Third Edition. Churchill Livingstone, New York, 1990. p 453.
22. Hustead, RF. BSS takes the sting out of local anesthesia. Ocular Surgery News 4:39;Nov 1986.
23. Gills JP, Loyd TL. A technique of retrobulbar block with paralysis of orbicularis oculi. Am Intra-ocular Implant Soc J 9:339-40;1983.
24. Davis DB II, Mandel MR. Posterior peribulbar anesthesia: An alternative to retrobulbar anesthesia. J Cataract Refract Surg 12:182-4;1986.
25. Bloomberg L. Administration of periocular anesthesia. J Cataract Refract Surg 12:677-9;1986.
26. Pautler SE, Grizzard WS. Blindness from retrobulbar injection into the optic nerve. Ophthalmic Surg 17:334-7;1986.
27. Carroll F, Roetth A Jr. The effect of retrobulbar injections of procaine on the optic nerve. Trans Am Acad Ophthalmol & Otolaryngol 356-65;May/June 1955.
28. Abelson MB, Mandel E. The effect of hyaluronidase on akinesia during cataract surgery. Ophthalmic Surg 20:325-6;1989.
29. Nicoll JMV, Treuren B, et al. Retrobulbar anesthesia: The role of hyaluronidase. Anesth Analg 65:1324-8;1986.
30. House PH, Hollands RH, Schulzer M. Choice of anesthetic agents for peribulbar anesthesia. J Cataract Refract Surg 17:80-3;1991.
31. Zahl K, Jordan A, et al. pH-adjusted bupivacaine and hyaluronidase for peribulbar block. Anesthesiology 72:230-2;1990.
32. Wang HS. Peribulbar anesthesia for ophthalmic procedures. J Cataract Refract Surg 14:441-3;1988.
33. Fleming JA, Byck R, Barash PG. Pharmacology and therapeutic applications of cocaine. Anesthesiology 73:518-31;1990.
34. Maier HW. Maier's Cocaine Addiction. Translated and edited by Kalant OJ. Addiction Research Foundation, Toronto, 1987 (original, 1926). pp 14-17.

35. McKay W, Morris R, Mushlin P. Sodium bicarbonate attenuates pain on skin infiltration with lidocaine, with or without epinephrine. Anesth Analg 66:572-4;1987.

36. Christoph R, Buchanan L, et al. Pain reduction in local anesthetic administration through pH buffering. Ann Emerg Med 17:117-20;1988.

37. Eccarius SG, Gordon ME, Parelman JJ. Bicarbonate-buffered lidocaine-epinephrine-hyaluronidase for eyelid anesthesia. Ophthalmology 97:1499-1501;1990.

38. Hustead, RF. Patent #4938970.

39. Hirschfelder AD, Bieter RN. Local anesthetics. Phys Rev 12:190-282;1932.

40. Ritchie JM, Ritchie B, Greengard P. The active structure of local anesthetics. J Pharmacol Exp Ther 150:152;1965.

41. Craig D, Habib G. Flaccid paraparesis following obstetrical epidural anesthesia: Possible role of benzyl alcohol. Anesth Analg 56:219-22;1977.

42. Marr WG, Wood R, et al. Effect of topical anesthetics on regeneration of corneal epithelium. Am J Ophthalmol 43:606-10;1957.

43. Maddi R, Concepcion M, et al. Evaluation of a new cutaneous topical anesthesia preparation. Reg Anesth 15:109-12;1990.

44. Maurice DM, Singh T. The absence of corneal toxicity with low-level topical anesthesia. Am J Ophthalmol 99:691-6;1985.

45. Moses RA (ed). Adler's Physiology of the Eye: Clinical Application, Seventh Edition. CV Mosby Co., St. Louis, 1981. pp78-82.

46. Caramel JP, Bonnel F, Rabischong P. The oculomotor nerve: biometry and endoneural fascicular systemization. Anat Clin 1983:5;159-68.

47. Bergen MP. Vascular Architechture in the Human Orbit. Swets & Zeitlinger B.V., Lisse, 1982.

48. de Jong RH. Physiology and Pharmacology of Local Anesthesia. Charles C. Thomas, Springfield, 1970. pp 82-95.

49a. de Jong RH. Local Anesthetics, Second Edition. Charles C. Thomas, Springfield, 1977. pp 51-62.

49b. ibid, p 98.

49c. ibid, p 108.

50a. Cousins MJ, Bridenbaugh PO (eds). Neural Blockade in Clinical Anesthesia and Management of Pain. JB Lippincott Co, Philadelphia, 1988. p 114.

50b. ibid, p 41.

51. O'Brien CS. Local anesthesia in ophthalmic surgery. Trans Sec Ophthalmology, AMA 237-52;1927.

52. Kasten GW. High serum bupivacaine concentrations produce rhythm disturbances similar to torsades de Pointes in anesthetized dogs. Reg Anesth 11:20-6;1986.

53. Albright GA. Cardiac arrest following regional anesthesia with etidocaine or bupivacaine. Anesthesiology 51:285-7;1979.

54. Zahl K, Nassif JM, et al. Simulated peribulbar injection of anesthetic. Ann Ophthalmol 23:114-7;1991.

55. Feibel RM. Robert E. Wright and the development of facial nerve akinesia. Surv Ophthalmol 33:523-8;1989.

56. Aldrete JA, Johnson DA. Evaluation of intracutaneous testing for investigation of allergy to local anesthetic agents. Anesth Analg 49:173-81;1970.

57. Schechter RJ. Management of inadvertent intraocular injections. Ann Ophthalmol 17:771-5;1985.

58. Foster AH, Carlson BM. Myotoxicity of local anesthetics and regeneration of the damaged muscle fibers. Anesth Analg 59:727-36;1980.

59. Rainin EA, Carlson BM. Postoperative diplopia and ptosis: A clinical hypothesis based on the myotoxicity of local anesthetics. Arch Ophthalmol 103:1337-9;1985.

60. Rao VA, Kawatra VK. Ocular myotoxic effects of local anesthetics. Can J Ophthalmol 23:171-3;1988.

61. de Faber JHN, von Noorden GK. Inferior rectus muscle palsy after retrobulbar anesthesia for cataract surgery. Am J Ophthalmol 112:209-11;1991.

62. Ankler-Moller E, Spangsberg N, et al. Subhypnotic doses of thiopentone and propofol cause analgesia to experimentally induced acute pain. Br J Anesthesia 66:185-188;1991.

Three

Robert F. Hustead, MD
Robert C. Hamilton, MB, BCh

TECHNIQUES

Background

This chapter contrasts the past techniques of ocular anesthesia with techniques advocated and in use by current writers. Anesthesia for cataract surgery and for enucleation will be emphasized—advances in technical knowledge in one area gradually lead to advances in application of technique in the other. For additional views, the reader is referred to "Regional Anesthesia for Intraocular Surgery" edited by Kenneth Zahl and Murray Meltzer in *The Ophthalmology Clinics of North America*, March 1990.

Historical Perspective

The demonstration that cocaine would effectively block painful sensation from the conjunctiva when instilled as a solution (instillation) or instilled as crystals (topical) ushered in a new era in ophthalmic surgery. Freedom from pain and cooperation on the part of the patient allowed the surgeon to remove diseased tissues and gave the eye a chance to heal.

However, topical cocaine did not diffuse deeply enough to abolish sensation from the iris in most patients and did not eliminate pain from pull on muscles or the cutting of the optic nerve. Additional injections (infiltration) of cocaine were needed to make the patient comfortable, or the surgeon was forced to operate with less than optimal conditions.

Most surgeons chose a subconjunctival infiltration of cocaine to decrease pain from pulling or cutting the iris in cataract surgery. The subconjunctival infiltration was rarely adequate to anesthetize the iris, so sedatives were added. Many patients continued to have pain, would close their eyes, or move at an inappropriate time.

With the addition of orbicularis akinesia by nerve block, introduced by Van Lint in 1914[1] and improved upon by Wright,[2] O'Brien,[3] and Atkinson,[4] it was possible to prevent patients from squinting or closing their eyes during cataract surgery even in the presence of pain. However, many would strain and move, and compromise the surgical field, even though they could not close their eyes. These conditions prevailed through 1920.

Enucleation with topical cocaine was extremely painful. Infiltration of the conjunctiva and along the muscles reduced the pain, but such infiltration through inflamed tissue was a time-consuming ordeal for patient and surgeon.[5,6,7]

Knapp,[8] in 1884, first described an injection of local anesthetic to block the ciliary nerves behind the eye (nerve block) to ease the pain of enucleation. The patient was not comfortable when the muscles and optic nerve were cut and became very pale and covered with cold sweat, which Knapp interpreted as "toxicity of cocaine in the vascular orbit." Therefore, Knapp believed that amounts of cocaine smaller than the volume he used were necessary (6 minims or 0.3 ml of 4%) for infiltration or nerve block in the orbit.

Injection of small volume did not render patients pain-free for enucleation because block of the ciliary nerves and pain fibers in the muscles was rarely effective at the recommended low volume of anesthetic since the nerves to the structures were not close. The majority of enucleations continued to be done under general anesthesia because neither topical plus infiltration nor topical plus nerve block was effective.

Because of the morbidity and poor operating conditions under general anesthesia, Elschnig and his assistant, Lowenstein, persisted in trying to achieve true anesthesia with local anesthetics for enucleation. They accomplished painless enucleation in 98% of patients using nerve block with cocaine and epinephrine, which they reported in 1908.[9] They used injections near the ciliary ganglion with resultant spread of anesthetic to the optic nerve sheath and the contiguous oculomotor and naso-ciliary nerves, along with injections in the orbit near the sensory nerves to the conjunctiva. They proved such a total block could be done with less than half the accepted toxic dose of cocaine.[9]

Their observation of patient calmness and freedom from pain led Duverger[7] to use the Prague method for enucleation. After observing the technique's effectiveness, he started using anesthetic injection in the area of the ciliary ganglion for patients in whom he expected difficulty with cataract surgery. It was blockade of the ciliary ganglion, ciliary nerves, and naso-ciliary nerve which led to freedom of pain from cataract surgery and better control of the eye during that procedure. Block of the facial nerve was a useful adjunct to prevent inadvertent eye closure and to decrease pressure of the muscles on the globe. Therefore, Elschnig and Duverger had established that perfect surgical conditions for cataract surgery were attained safely by regional block, then called ciliary ganglion block.

Atkinson[4] and SR Gifford[10] realized that freedom of pain, akinesia of the lids and globe, and the lowered intraocular pressure of ciliary ganglion block during cataract surgery gave a much higher incidence of excellent surgical results by those who had adopted the technique.[7,11,12] Therefore, Atkinson encouraged ciliary ganglion block by cone injection, facial block, and globe paresis for cataract surgery in the United States and updated his technique every three years.[4,13-21] Freedom from pain because of cone block of the ciliary nerves and good surgical results led to the explosion of cataract surgery of the 1940s and 50s. Nonetheless, some patients still had pain and would strain at the wrong time from inadequate anesthesia, and some globes did not become akinetic. This led some surgeons to adopt the apical injection of H. Gifford,[22] but many simply added more local anesthetic.

The use of higher volumes of local anesthetic for cone injection to produce ciliary ganglion block and oculomotor akinesia plus oculocompression[23] to reduce vitreous volume and orbital volume led to an even higher incidence of good surgical results. Good surgical conditions provided an operative field suitable for lens implantation.

Therefore, akinesia of the lids and the ocular muscles, anesthesia of the orbit and the globe, and hypotony of the globe became the desired anesthetic outcomes for cataract surgery in the 1970s.

These desired conditions provided totally painless enucleation and established that injections of local anesthetic in the orbit eliminate pain in the orbit and globe.

It took ophthalmology about 100 years to accomplish reliable, excellent results with local anesthesia by abandoning four false concepts generated during the birth of local anesthesia in ophthalmology: (1) the use of small volume local anesthetic injection in the orbit, (2) the placement of needles shallow in the orbit or along the muscles to block eye pain, (3) the avoidance of pressure over the globe after pre-anesthetic injection and needle withdrawal, and (4) incising as soon as the needle was withdrawn. When these techniques were eliminated, painless cataract surgery and enucleation were possible with local anesthesia.

Between 1760 and 1960, successful cataract surgery meant that the patient regained some useful vision with cataract spectacles. Cataract surgery was usually postponed until patients were almost blind. An unsuccessful surgery resulted in vision loss or blindness which would have been the the patient's condition if surgery was not performed. Therefore, the occasional loss of vision or blindness was insignificant when compared to the safe, excellent surgical results that could be provided to many patients by cataract surgery with local anesthesia. The greater safety of local anesthesia was accepted, although enucleation was more often done with general.

From 1950 through the 1970s there was much interest in making cone injection of the ciliary ganglion even more reliable, establishing the safety of the amide local anesthetics for blocks, and developing longer lasting blocks for less painful, less risky post-operative care.[24] There was a rapid surge in ophthalmic diagnosis and the modalities that could be treated, and a concomitant geometric increase in the use of cone injection to inject therapeutic drugs and prevent pain from the rapidly proliferating glaucoma and retinal procedures. The block was being done often; its name was shortened to "retrobulbar block."

However, in the early 1970s, reports of death on the operating table from a combination of sedation and local anesthesia led to a re-examination of the use of heavy sedation with local during cataract surgery. The accepted benefits of heavy sedation to decrease the danger of the CNS toxicity of local anesthetic drugs was no longer valid. Since large volume local anesthetic injection in the orbit rendered the orbit insensitive to pain and allowed patient cooperation, sedation was a poor excuse for the use of toxic amounts of epinephrine, inadequate blocks, or uncomfortable surgical carts.

In the 1970s and '80s, references appeared describing the risks of injury to the optic nerve or globe from cone injections and brainstem apnea from large volume injections. What had been accepted as a totally safe procedure was now questioned by practitioners and attorneys. Some of the reports incriminated the use of disposable ultra-sharp needles introduced during the 1960s, others incriminated the procedure. Nobody questioned the mechanical dexterity, the training of those making such injections, or the anatomic subtleties of safe technique, and no university had examined the principles or the results of teaching cone or sub-Tenon's injections, or subcapsular block to ophthalmology residents. There were no data comparing the incidence of learning curve injuries for those teaching the technique nor any good data on teaching methods or curriculum.

Unfortunately, at about the same time, some ophthalmologists began training other personnel to perform the cone injection. It was suggested in reports that part of the increase in injury of the 1980s was due to non-ophthalmologists doing the blocks.[3-25]

Semantics

From the foregoing historical perspective, the reader may be a bit confused about terminology for anesthetic technique for good reason, it is confusing. The authors have tried to avoid conflicting terminology by eliminating the vernacular and putting quotations marks around "cliches." This area could be improved by authoritative definitions, etymology, or anatomic neurologic nomenclature.

Topical anesthesia originally implied the placing of cocaine crystals in the cul-de-sac or on the globe. Instillation anesthesia was the placing of a solution of local anesthetic in the conjunctival sac or on the cornea. Today topical refers to instillation of solution or crystals (rarely used anymore).

Infiltration anesthesia was the injection of local anesthetic in the subcutaneous tissues or between tissue planes to distend that plane and fill it with local anesthetic to block all the nerves which traversed the plane. Nerve block referred to making an injection alongside or in the fascial plane of major nerves. Atkinson referred to Knapp's technique as the first retrobulbar nerve block.[19,21] Dr. Knapp referred to his own technique as "injection of local anesthetic close to the posterior surface of the eye into the area of the ciliary nerves close to the globe." Using 0.3 ml of anesthetic, he obviously was trying to anesthetize the tiny ciliary nerves just before they entered the eye. Knapp put forceps on the globe, and withdrew the globe until he could put a needle behind it. Atkinson refers to this first retrobulbar block as producing "retrobulbar anesthesia" for painless enucleation. Dr. Knapp indicates the operation caused pain during division of the muscles and the optic nerve.

Therefore, neither historically, nor by procedure description, nor by effect should Knapp be considered as the originator of "retrobulbar anesthesia," if "retrobulbar anesthesia" is the term of the 1960s attached to blocks of the ciliary ganglion, the naso-ciliary nerve, and the oculomotor nerve as described by Atkinson, Duverger, Gifford, or Lowenstein. Knapp is perhaps the father of cocaine-facilitated globe forceps fixation to allow "retrobulbar infiltration."

A number of authors purposely infiltrated local anesthetic behind the eye or along the muscles for enucleation; they tried to fill the space with anesthetic. They were all making "retrobulbar" infiltration; several reported "painless" surgery with this technique, although the technique induced significant pain and was considered by most surgeons as neither practical nor reliable.[7]

Lowenstein and Elschnig deserve credit for placing a needle in an area to block the ciliary ganglion, the ciliary nerves, and the oculomotor nerve to produce good conditions for enucleation. However, even they additionally infiltrated the area of sensory nerves to the conjunctiva and orbit for completeness of anesthesia and patient comfort. A ciliary ganglion block or a cone block alone does not provide anesthesia for comfortable enucleation. Atkinson referred to his block as a "retrobulbar injection into the muscular cone or cone injection."[4,21]

A retrobulbar injection is any injection behind the equator of the eye in which the needle lies behind the projection of the equator—even 1 degree inclination of the needle toward the optical axis from the equator of the eye places it in the "retrobulbar space." The anesthesia produced by bulk flow of anesthetics within such a retrobulbar space could be considered retrobulbar anesthesia. All sensory nerves to the globe and orbit and all motor nerves to the extraocular muscles are in the retrobulbar space, and therefore must be blocked there to eliminate the pain of enucleation.

It would be convenient if the space behind the eye were limited by a membrane linking each of the rectus muscles to its neighbor, and thus define a "retrobulbar, intermuscular," and intraconal space. No such structure exists, and therefore a retrobulbar space exists that includes the optic nerve and all of the rectus muscles and all the tissue between them and the periorbit. It can be divided by a true cone of muscles in the posterior orbit into intraconal and extraconal compartments.

In the posterior orbit, the rectus muscles converge sufficiently to unite each to the other to form a retrobulbar conal space. Atkinson rightfully described the opening of that space as a site to inject local anesthetics to produce cone anesthesia. Cone injection is very logical terminology, and he produced retrobulbar anesthesia by blocking the ciliary ganglion and the ciliary nerves within the muscular cone and akinesia or paresis by anesthetic spread to the motor nerves. He described a specific retrobulbar block.

However, there are many other retrobulbar areas into which anesthetic can be injected to produce retrobulbar anesthesia; some areas may or may not block the abducens, oculomotor, or trochlear nerves, but will produce anesthesia.

An injection of local anesthetic outside the retrobulbar space could be logically called a peribulbar or periocular injection, instead of periorbial. But, if one injects anesthetic in this area and ends up with ocular akinesia or ocular anesthesia, one has made a "peribulbar/periocular" injection to produce retrobulbar akinesia or anesthesia; posterior injections produce orbital or retrobulbar anesthesia.

But what are the confines of the periorbital space into which the injections travel anteriorly or posteriorly? What historical or etymological precedent exists for re-defining the periorbital space as an anterior or posterior peribulbar or periocular space, when anesthetics injected there produce retrobulbar anesthesia?

There is no anatomic or etymological precedent for the term periocular or peribulbar anesthesia. Periocular injection, according to the diagrams of Bloomberg, should cause anesthetic to arrive at the sensory nerves to the eyelid and to block the small fibers of the facial nerve pre-septally that go the orbicularis muscle. It thus produced periocular anesthesia of the anterior orbit. However, if it produced ocular anesthesia or orbital akinesia, it has done so by anesthetic entering the retrobulbar space by bulk spread or diffusion to block the nerves in the retrobulbar space.

It is convenient for physicians to use a phrase to define a new technique, to make it easy for the general medical audience to make a transition from one procedure to another. However, use of terminology which is anatomically or pharmacologically misleading should not continue in the subsequent literature.

The authors suggest that the term retrobulbar anesthesia continue to signify the blockade of nerves traversing the retrobulbar space; whether those nerves are intraconal or extraconal could be signified by the addition of those descriptors. The authors believe that injections should be named as to the site of needle entrance and the location of the point of the needle, and that anesthesia should be defined by the area where the nerves are blocked. Thus, an attempt to block the frontal nerve in the periorbital space above the levator muscle would be called a retrobulbar extraconal block of the frontal nerve.

Therefore, currently used injections termed peribulbar or periocular should be referred to descriptively: anterior retrobulbar injections or anterior periorbital injections, depending upon where the needle point is actually located (see Figure 1.59a-i). This would suffice to draw attention to the fact that the technique disallows placing needles in the posterior orbit where damage to deep orbital structures is anatomically possible and that the anesthetist knows the needle point locus.

For example, injections of anesthetic between the equator of the eye and the hind surface of the globe could be called anterior retrobulbar injections. Mid-orbital injections are those planned behind the hind surface, but anterior to the cone; cone injection or ciliary ganglion block (its historical term) are those injections in the cone; and posterior retrobulbar or apical injections are those with needle placement in the orbital apex. Site of injection is thus delineated exactly.

Anterior diffusion from the orbit can produce orbicularis akinesia. Local anesthetic arrives in the pre-septal space by injection, bulk spread, diffusion, or a combination. Needle entrance, path, and point location require many words. Description of the resulting anesthesia, analgesia, paresis, and akinesia also requires many words. Perhaps clarity and brevity are best served by the use of eponyms—Atkinson '34,[4] Atkinson '65,[21] Gills/Loyd '83,[26] Johnson/Gills '90,[27] Davis/Mandel '86,[28] Davis/Mandel '90,[29] Bloomberg '86,[30] Bloomberg '91,[31] or Wang '88[32] technique.

Since the dura splits into two layers at the entrance of the optic nerve with the parietal dura becoming the periorbit, and the visceral layer of dura covering the optic nerve becoming the optic sheath continuing forward as Tenon's capsule, it makes sense to refer to any block between the orbital apex and the orbital septum as an orbital epidural block. This calls attention to the site of block, knowledge base required, risks of the technique, and skill level expected.

Needles and Usage

Needles come in a variety of lengths, wall thickness or gauge, point style, and keenness (Figure 3.1). A relatively small number of needles have found their way into regional anesthesia of the orbit (Figure 3.1).

As the wall thickness and the amount of metal in the wall are reduced, all needles become flexible; special alloys make needles malleable. Malleable needles have never found much use in ophthalmology, except as tear duct probes.

Almost all needles in current use are made of stainless steel, the type chosen varying with the manufacturer and the specific mechanical means used to form the needle. Varying the additive compounds in stainless steel can make needles of extraordinary keenness and extraordinary resistance to bending or fracture; however, the steel must be ductile to allow the tube blank to be formed into small needles. Ductility and the ability to make a keen point are mutually exclusive except by expensive metallurgical endeavors. Therefore, manufacturers usually settle for a compromise, which limits the keenness of points and makes needles unnecessarily flexible.

When a tube of stainless steel is ground to make a point, the more shallow the angle of grind, the less force required for the needle point to penetrate a tissue such as skin. The longer the point, the easier to make a sharp point. The longest bevels commonly used are 12°; needles can be ground as much as 45°. Such short bevels are often used to obtain cores of tissue for pathological examination. Coring needles are partly a factor of the degree of the bevel grind, but mostly the gauge of the tubing.

The needle is called a flat grind needle after the primary grind is made. Flat grind needles have a very sharp conical edge with limited penetrating qualities. The needle will usually go into skin one-half to one-third the way up the bevel of the needle with minimal force, making a crescent cut, but the side edge of the needle has no keen edge so the tissue is stretched to allow needle passage, if it passes. More commonly a core of tissue enters the shaft by compression, plugs the needle and is amputated by the sharp heel of the needle.

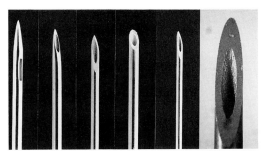

Figure 3.1a. Bevel view of needles used in ophthalmology magnified at 15 x. Left to right 30 gauge, 27 gauge, 25 gauge Atkinson' or Straus, 25 gauge, Thornton, 25 gauge Galindo Pinpoint, and 23 gauge flat ground needle. (Photo courtesy Charles Cooley, University of Kansas, Wichita.)

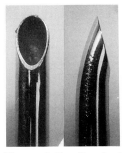

Figure 3.1b. Bevel view of Hustead 18 gauge epidural needle. (Photo courtesy Doug Mastel, Mastel Instruments, Rapid City. SD)

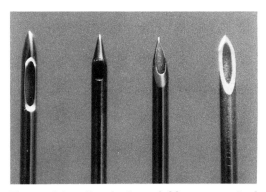

Figure 3.1c. Bevel view of 22 gauge spinal needles at 8x. Left to right—Sprotte, Whitacre, Greene, and Quinke.

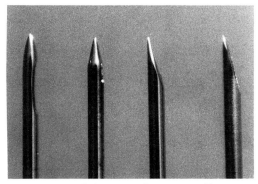

Figure 3.1d. Side view of same needles as in 3.1c. (Figures 3.1c and d Courtesy Cheryl Dixon, MD University of Florida College of Medicine, Gainsville, FL and Becton-Dickinson, Rutherford, NJ).

To make a needle that will penetrate skin easily without coring, additional faces are cut by compound grinding. If enough additional faces on the needle are ground and all are finished, it will have an extremely fine, sharp point that will allow the needle to make a nearly flat incision that readily stretches to admit the needle with minimum coring. The point will readily bend if it contacts any rigid structures, producing a barb.

The shallower the primary grind and the shallower the compound grinding, the shorter the needle bevel and the more abuse the point will take. Short beveled needles can be filled with stylets to prevent coring. These are made to enter the subarachnoid space where the short bevel can be placed entirely in the CSF and no core of tissue introduced there.[33] Such needles leave a gaping wound. Injection must be made intermittently or continuously to clear the needle to prevent core compression when used without a stylet. Atkinson designed a short beveled 23 gauge needle with a single compound grind for cone block; it readily penetrates for half the bevel length, but resists full penetration because of coring; it leaves a gaping scleral or retinal wound.

Long beveled needles were desirable to make intramuscular or subcutaneous injections to enter the skin and muscles with very little force to make a tiny opening, and to allow the anesthetic or solution to exit the needle over a wide area. The needle point barbs easily; as disposable needles they are kind to patients. Such needles can be used to inject local anesthetics, but the needle point can enter tissue a distance from the area of injection and fail to dissect in the desired plane, but cause damage.

The smaller the needle, the shorter the bevel can be while maintaining a keen point. Modern 27 gauge needles have a shorter bevel than short beveled 23 gauge needles (Figure 3.1). Keenness can be improved by polishing the point as in the Thornton needle.

The smaller the diameter of the needle (the higher the gauge number), the less critical the point of the needle to penetrate the skin, until at 34 gauge, needles hardly need a point. However, 34 gauge needles are so flexible that it is hard to insert them any distance; they bend on entering the epidermis.

Compound needles have been made with extremely fine points and a progressively larger shaft, so that a very fine needle point could be used to introduce the needle with the shaft stiff enough to allow the needle to travel through tissue by expanding it. This is the design of the common sewing needle or pin, which is very cheaply produced. A "pinpoint" hollow needle with the opening on the side has been introduced into ophthalmology (Figure 3.1a).

Needles with a taper or pin point are also called "atraumatic" needles because they stretch rather than cut tissue. These needles are commonly used in cardiovascular and intestinal surgery because they can force themselves through tissues without actually cutting, and a suture can follow with very little leakage around the needle entry point. Taper point hollow needles are very expensive to manufacture. They core more readily than bevel point needles and are used in micro tissue sampling.

Coring can also be prevented by bending the tubing to 15-30° and grinding the point flat to the shaft—the "Huber point"® needle invented for non-coring intradermal injection is an example. Such needles are mostly used in epidural anesthesia in much larger gauge to pass a catheter out at a slight angle to facilitate placing the catheter in the epidural space (Figure 3.1b).

Both the length and the diameter of a needle affect the amount of pressure required to cause a given volume of solution to flow in a given period of time. Conversely, the longer the needle and the smaller the diameter, the less fluid will go out per unit of time for a given size syringe. Flow in the very small needles, although they are capillary tube in dimension, often becomes turbulent if sufficient force is supplied.

After World War I, the best needles were made out of steel/platinum/iridium alloys. These needles maintained a reasonably keen point only as long as they were ground and finished properly and polished. Polishing the edge of razors or needles is best done by stropping with leather. Thus by a combination of grinding, polishing, and stropping, platinum iridium needles could be made extremely sharp though the points would dull with one touch of cartilage or bone. High quality stainless steel became the standard during the 1930s. These needles took a keen point with stropping which they would retain through many uses.

Disposable Needles

A tremendous incentive for the development of disposable needles arose after World War II when the armed services needed to keep needles sterile in the field. The manufacturing skills had been established in Germany and were imported to this country. Hospitals were eager to replace their older needles with a disposable product, especially if that product saved them money.

Some of the disposable needles were superior to the single use needles they replaced; however, some were of very poor quality. The industry has become highly competitive, and it behooves the practitioner to select for quality since the price will most likely be competitive.

The relationship between length and diameter of the needle was established by the example of Braun in 1904 for carbon steel needles[34a] to allow the smallest needle shaft that would penetrate skin without flexing when the point was keen.

Thus the 27 gauge 10 mm needle, the 25 gauge 25 mm needle, the 24 gauge 30 mm needle, the 23 gauge 35 mm needle, the 22 gauge 60 to 90 mm needle, the 21 gauge 100 mm needle, and the 20 gauge 125 mm needle were produced. A 50 mm needle was made by cutting a 60 mm needle, grinding it, and making a new point.

Few anesthesiologists or ophthalmologists currently use re-usable needles. The mass produced disposable needles have been a blessing to many patients and the reliability of their manufacture has been a boon to anesthesia providers. However, there are occasional reject needles with mass produced needles just as there used to be problems in self-sharpening. One needs to know what one expects of his tool and to avoid using a defective tool.

One problem with the smaller gauge disposable needles is that about 1% are duller than they should be, and occasionally the shafts have not been sufficiently polished or siliconized to allow them to glide through tissues. The wary professional will simply discard those needles.

The second disadvantage of the smaller gauge keen needles is that when they are allowed to touch bone or tough ligamentous tissue, the points rapidly dull or barb so they are less serviceable for doing blocks in which the needle is introduced a given distance to contact bone, then retracted and redirected.

The clear polypropylene hub disposable needles which allow a volume of 0.01 ml of blood to be visible in the hub are immensely beneficial to techniques which touch or enter areas of blood vessels. The authors use the 27 and 30 gauge clear hub needles for all ophthalmic anesthesia.

Choice of Needle Length

The stainless steel re-usable needles were made with a very high quality stainless steel that was more resilient to bending and breaking than the current disposable needles. Their shafts were highly polished and the points were of quality metal that would take repeated honing. Unfortunately, flexion at the solder joint or weld between the hub of the needle and the shaft often occurred, which when straightened more than a given number of times, led to breakage at that point. Therefore, in regional anesthesia it was considered poor technique to approach the skin with the hub of the needle because the needle could break off in the skin (the same can happen to disposable needles).

As a result, one chose needles of a length suitable to go the distance expected, plus five millimeters. The shaft size was that which would allow the point to penetrate the tissues of the path without flexing the shaft and which would allow the desired flow rate of anesthetic as the force required doubled with a needle twice as long.

It is pleasing to look at historical treatises on ophthalmic regional anesthesia and see the hub of Braun needles or Labat needles projected from the skin of the orbit by five millimeters, attesting to the background of those who were using them. It is even more satisfying to see such concepts in current ophthalmic presentations.[32]

It is very common in current treatises on ophthalmic anesthesia to see the hub of a needle pressing skin and depression of the skin with the hub for 3 to 20 mm before injection of anesthetic takes place.

Therefore, choice of needle length in ophthalmology is obviously no longer dependent upon the distance to the site of injection plus five millimeters, but a measure of the stretch of the skin. This could lead to a disconcerting retrieval should a needle break. However, pushing against the skin with a needle has another ominous side.

When the hub of the needle presses against skin, the tension subtracts tactile discrimination from the operator so that it is difficult to sense that the point of the needle is making contact with deeper structures. Inadvertent damage to nerves and blood vessels is more likely, just as it is more likely that dull needles will cause more trauma or undeserved penetration of structures than will sharp needles. How is this possible?

Dull vs. Sharp Point Needles

The polished stainless steel needles or siliconized needles flow through tissues if the point is keen enough to make a track—then slight touch will allow the operator to identify layers or structures during passage. Dull needles do not allow the shaft to flow through adipose or muscle tissue and lead to flexing of the shaft with contact with minor adipose tissue septa or muscle. Contact would give false information about the presence of a significant septum or structure. Thrusting the needle to penetrate the impediment then provides inertia leading to penetration of an adjacent structure without "feeling" it.

Furthermore, the dull needle will cause the "bent arrow" effect. When the needle contacts connective tissue, the shaft will bend in the plane of the bevel opening before penetration is complete; when an additional thrust is made to push the needle through, the needle point will then veer off in an angle from where it touched the structure, thus not following a true course. The more flexible the needle, the more likely there will be deviation.

When short beveled dull needles are used, for instance to identify the epidural space and allow entrance without cutting the dura (please see Figure 3.1b), a sharp needle was intended to be placed at the ligaments and connective tissue to make a tunnel, followed by the dull needle following the exact track of the sharp needle until it would impinge upon ligamentum flavum. A similar technique would be necessary in the orbit to assure safety if it were necessary to put needles in the orbital apex with a millimeter of tolerance.

The use of dull needles to reduce danger to orbital apex structures from cone injection is debatable, it is even more controversial in the mid-orbit. Atkinson's early papers (1934, 1936, 1943, and 1948) did not suggest using dull needles to avoid damaging structures in the orbit; used was the Labat 35 mm (a 25 gauge sharp needle in 1934), and then BD needles afterward. Atkinson emphasized replacing needles in their carriers to maintain sharpness.

In 1948, Gifford published his first paper inserting a 50 mm needle into the orbital apex and using a needle with the cutting edge buffed off to reduce retrobulbar hemorrhage. Since dull needles reduced Gifford's[22b] incidence of hemorrhage from 5% to 1% the concept may have been borrowed by Atkinson. Only from 1955 on did Atkinson's papers advise use of a dull point needle—one made by BD to his specifications (35 mm flat grind 18° bevel needle). The needle has a wedge cutting tip with single compound grind to allow insertion through skin (please see Figure 3.1). It was a far cry from the buffered round point needle of Gifford and is a far cry from the "Atkinson disposable needles"—the design patent has probably expired. One percent is better than 5% retrobulbar hemorrhage, but even Lowenstein had only 0.6% with sharp needles, and most of them were early in the method.

Lowenstein's descriptions clearly indicate inserting a Braun needle without a syringe into the orbital apex so that he could feel with the needle as the needle by-passed structures. Such delicate touch and feel are not a part of the province of all persons, but should be for ophthalmologists doing delicate surgery.

Infiltration vs. Orbital Nerve Block in the Orbit

Attaching a needle to a syringe to inject as the needle is traveling is a technique known as infiltration anesthesia; it was the technique of choice to push blood vessels away from the needle as it was forced through subcutaneous tissue for infiltration of large volumes of anesthetic under the skin. The operator expects to feel nothing during infiltration techniques, and infiltration stops when a delicate area is reached that requires feel of structures. At such structures the syringe is removed or at least infiltration is stopped so the fingers can sense structures until the needle is located in the proper place; the needle is then cleared of cored material if coring needles are used.

Infiltration in the delicate structures of the orbit would have emptied the 2 ml syringe of those days, with possible needle impalement of delicate structures with no feedback. The duller the point, the less one can feel. Infiltration might have been beneficial through the capsulo-palpebral fascia area or past the equator of the eye. From that point on, delicate structure technique should have been encouraged, and careful placement of the needle point a given measured distance from a given reference point. Test injections to clear the needle and tests for intravascular placement were then indicated.

It is not surprising that Gifford, using a sharp needle and injecting as the needle advanced into an enclosed space, would eventually impinge an artery against bone or tendon without feeling the impingement and lacerate the vessel. What is surprising is that Gifford, a superb scientist, should attribute the reduction of hemorrhage in his technique solely to the switch to the buffed round point needle. Could it not have been just the learning curve for his technique since the reduction of hemorrhage from 5% to 1% is very compatible with the mastery of a technical skill—and perhaps the unconscious effort not to introduce the needle quite so far into the blind area where all the bleeding originated?

Damage from Needles

The laws of penetration of structures with needles have not changed. A needle that penetrates the skin will penetrate an artery, vein, nerve, dura, or sclera providing the structure cannot move away from the needle, such as the ophthalmic vein and the optic nerve in the apex or with the globe in a forced position of gaze or retracted by fingers. The force required to penetrate the skin is a product of the diameter of the needle and the shape and keenness of its cutting surface.

The penetration forces of the skin are similar to the penetration forces of the sclera. As the needle advances through either structure, force of penetration is counter-acted by the strain on the structure. The skin gives a certain distance before being penetrated. Contact with bulbar capsulo-palpebral fascia causes the globe to move before it is penetrated. When the globe or the skin is free to move, the distance either travels before a needle penetrates it is a function of the strain on the elements that oppose the motion and the contact angle.

Galindo et al have recently measured penetration forces of the skin and sclera and found them almost identical at any penetration speed (Table 3.1);[36] the penetration force of a 25 gauge Atkinson needle was almost identical for a regular 25 gauge sharp point.[36] One of the authors did similar experiments before doing his first retrobulbar block. It is true that the sclera in very myopic eyes may be quite attenuated and more easily penetrated than skin, but the reciprocal is also true. Therefore, the astute clinician examines the skin and the nature of the globe before putting a needle close to either—and then DOES NOT put a needle close to the sclera or optic nerve.

Prevention of injury to or penetration of a structure is best attained by avoiding that structure (the globe, optic nerve) or by paralleling the course of the structure (the globe, arteries, optic nerve).

If one wishes to reduce hemorrhage from inadvertent contact with a vessel, one reduces the diameter of the cutting edge that will approach it. One can penetrate any artery with a 30 gauge needle at a 45° angle, withdraw the needle, and rarely will there be hemorrhage through the adventitia of that vessel. Penetrating the same vessel with a 22 gauge needle causes a column of blood to spurt one foot at 120 mmHg and one meter at 180 mmHg.

Ophthalmologists use these principles when they introduce a 30 or 27 gauge needle through clear cornea and expect the wound to self-seal. If one is impinging upon an artery with a needle that will penetrate the skin, then hemorrhage will be proportional to the size of the hole made by the point of the needle, to the shape of the hole which is made by the point, and to the hydrostatic pressure. Crescent holes from short beveled flat grind needles seal poorly and can lead to major hemorrhage.

If one uses the dull point to signal contact with an artery, it is as likely to induce hemorrhage as approaching that same artery with a sharp needle because the force required to move the dull needle through adjacent structures is much greater and more inertia is developed. However, if the artery is approached at a 5 to 10° angle, it will be very difficult to penetrate it even with the sharpest of points, providing the bevel faces the artery. The bevel will allow a flexible needle to parallel the structure instead of penetrating it.

The incidence of hemorrhage is a function of the size and shape of the point which enters the blood vessel. Damage is proportional to the surface area of the dissecting surface—about 5X for a 22 gauge compared to a 25 gauge. Substitution of a 22 gauge dull needle sharp enough to penetrate the skin would not diminish the damage compared to a 25 gauge needle that would also barely penetrate the skin.

Choice of Needle Gauge and Point

The smallest gauge needle possible for the given length of tissue to be traversed by a point of certain keenness is the optimal choice in regional anesthesia because the smaller the needle, the less damage to the structure. Tactile discrimination is learned by choosing a needle point and gauge suited to the task and be as constant as possible in technique so that feedback from the point is reliable.

The force for injection increases to maintain flow at a constant rate as the diameter decreases and almost doubles with each gauge size. When it is important to limit flow to decrease pain of injection or prevent CNS cardiac catastrophe, it is wise to match syringe size, needle length and gauge. Even signs like "slow injection" mean different things. A 3 ml syringe and a 30 gauge 1″ needle makes an almost perfect combination—1 ml/10 seconds with moderate finger pressure. A 5 ml syringe and a 1 1/4″ 27 gauge needle allows for larger flow (1 ml/7 seconds). Remember that injection in the orbit at a rate faster than 1 ml/20 seconds causes pain. Unfortunately, most inject as fast as possible because they have not been patients themselves.

The optimal shape of the point and cutting quality of the point are still moot. The needle point should be able to penetrate the skin and conjunctiva easily, pass through minor septa without causing diplopia, and allow the septa to slide along the needle shaft. Additionally it should signal proximity to the condensed tissue of nerves, arteries, veins, dura, or sclera.

The length of the bevel opening of the needle is important in terms of damage to structures should the entire bevel be placed within that structure. A short bevel needle is much more likely to cause intra-arterial or sub-arachnoid injection, or intra-neural damage. With a longer bevel needle, the point may enter the structure, but fluid will flow out the posterior aspect of the bevel and not cause infiltration damage.

Short beveled needles are mandatory when trying to enter the subarachnoid space and are contraindicated in the posterior orbit with a straight needle or in the mid-orbit with a curved needle where they might enter the subarachnoid space and cause the entire injection to flow into that compartment.

Short beveled fine needles are more likely to bow and to deviate from the intended linear path, whereas keen fine needles are more likely to continue in a straight path. Either can signal contact with a structure if the operator is attentive. Both can contact a structure and not penetrate it.

The secret is to have the bevel face the structure at an angle approximating the bevel opening to prevent digging in, 18 to 25° for most short beveled needles, but 15° for standard needles. Thus a short bevel may give 3 to 10° of extra safety (0.1 mm), if it does not cause a gaping hole.

Bevel to The Globe

It is considered safer to have the bevel of the needle face the globe as a needle approaches the equator and passes beyond it. If the angle of the bevel is such that the heel of the bevel opening will touch the surface before the point, the point will tend not to dig in. This same logic was first applied to linear structures,[37] such as the periosteum, muscles, arteries, or the subarachnoid space. Contact with any structure should signal the operator *to withdraw the length of the bevel*, turn the needle 90° to ascertain absence of flow of blood or fluid, withdraw the needle to an area where the tissues are free, and change the angle so the subsequent course may clear the structure.

Changes in Needle Angle

In regional anesthesia technique, it is common to touch the needle to the periosteum or ligament to note depth. The needle then is always retracted to the subcutaneous tissues before change of angle is made—the depth marker being set at the point of contact.

In 1955, Atkinson made major changes in his recommended anesthesia technique involving change of angle. Prior to 1955, the needle was shown leaving the skin site of entry at the inferior orbital rim, passing between the inferior and lateral rectus muscles and proceeding toward the orbital apex to stop at the opening of the muscle cone.

In 1955, the technique was changed to have the needle go in an inferior direction to touch the floor of the orbit to give more clearance and locate the equator. Then the needle direction was changed by pushing on the syringe to take the needle supero-nasally in its path to the orbital apex. Geometry and anatomy make this technique confusing and anatomy makes it potentially dangerous.

One expects that the needle could be directed from its inferior direction past the equator of the eye by depressing the syringe so that the shaft would go true in a new direction toward the apex. Bendable needles may not do this. They may go in the intended new direction or many other angles depending upon where a point of fulcrum lies with respect to the applied forces. It is very important to have the needle point in free tissue before changing direction so there is no fulcrum to give a false passage.

It is possible that more than one globe has been perforated by persons using this change of direction technique. The point of the needle with the bevel facing the globe would tend to dig into the periosteum of the maxillary sinus; when the syringe was depressed, the needle point would not necessarily free up. The anesthetist would then either press harder on the syringe, be unable to free the needle point, and would retract the syringe while pushing downward which would inadvertently put the needle anterior to the equator of the eye. Thinking he had clearance, the anesthetist would perforate the globe. Flexible needles cannot be expected to change direction in denser capsulo-palpebral fascia.

Walking the floor of the orbit is not recommended because the maxillary sinus is irregular, mucocles can be entered, and false passage into the infraorbital canal or inferior fissure can occur.

Technical Perspective

Today, with uniformly keen needles with small shaft diameter and choice of points, it is possible to choose a needle of given length and appropriate gauge to minimize damage to structures, to enter the skin without needle flexing, and to provide maximum tactile discrimination. Needle length chosen should avoid the hub touching the skin. Longer than necessary needles are more flexible and cause patients fear.

Shorter needles are less flexible and allow faster injection. Use of shorter than optimal length to give a pretense of safety and allow faster injection SHOULD NOT be confused with optimal technique. Rate of injection should be matched to patient comfort and safety.

Special needles are available and require new learning and skills and judgements. We cannot recommend them until they have been better tested in a prospective randomized trial with operators of various skill levels.

Oculocompression

A major advance in orbital anesthesia occurred when Kirsch reported better conditions for intracapsular cataract surgery with five minutes of deliberate pressure over the orbital tissues with the fingers to produce hypotony of the globe and diminish vitreous volume.[38] A few authors previously mentioned that conditions seemed better if digital massage was done after the block and before the surgery started because the anesthetic spread better.[4,38]

Once established that some digital pressure was beneficial, the next questions became how much and how long. Various authors believed that 30 seconds on and five seconds off would allow good retinal perfusion,[23] other authors determined that continuous pressure could be maintained much longer at low pressure without retinal damage.[39] Therefore, time chosen should be that to produce optimum results without injury. These guidelines have not been established.

A number of devices have been designed to make the technique more accurate and reproducible and to free up personnel from the task. Such devices include the Oculopressor®[38], the mercury bag, the Honan balloon,®[40] the nerf ball, the Super Pinky®, and the bulb of an irrigation syringe held in place by an elastic band.[41] The design features, advantages and disadvantages of each of these devices are different, and all seem to give excellent results in the hands of those familiar with them. The Oculopressor® and the Honan balloon® have the advantage of giving a manometric readout of applied pressure, and some relationship can be made when they are used between the amount of applied pressure and the time and pressure over which orbital and ocular decompression become optimum.

There is good evidence that five minutes of digital compression or oculopressor time is highly beneficial in reducing vitreous volume;[23] that 10 minutes is better,[42] and that 20 minutes is best in terms of producing ocular hypotony.[43] Orbital decompression precedes or occurs along with reduction of vitreous volume.[42]

To obtain a soft eye and orbital space for intracapsular or extracapsular extraction with lens implantation, one should count on 20 minutes of orbital decompression using the Honan device at a pressure of 20 to 25 mmHg applied pressure; a few patients will require more. Some practitioners use more pressure for longer periods of time with no suggestion of retinal damage.

The dynamics of oculocompression are still moot. However, the effect is quite dramatic and highly beneficial. An injection of local anesthetic sufficient to fill the superior lid crease will keep the orbit distended and intraocular pressure elevated for upwards of 20 minutes if no attempt is made to massage the globe. If, however, 20 mmHg orbital pressure is exerted by the Honan balloon or a similar device for five minutes, the orbit in more than 50% of persons will be decompressed to a volume less than before the injection was made, and intraocular pressure will be below control. However, a few orbits will require 20 minutes to reduce to that volume. The slow to soften orbits are often associated with obese faces, diabetes, Graves' disease, and prednisone therapy. If the device is left in place long enough, all orbits will eventually reduce to equal or less than their volume prior to the injection of anesthetic in the orbit.

Many who use oculocompression devices believe that hyaluronidase in the anesthetic mixture accentuates the rate at which the orbit decompresses on average and minimizes the number of patients who are slow to decompress.

On the other hand, the reduction of intraocular pressure does not necessarily follow the reduction in orbital volume, either in time or extent of reduction. It is not uncommon for intraocular pressure to be at or below normal in five minutes in an orbit that is still full of fluid. Likewise, it is not uncommon for an orbit to be totally decompressed in five minutes, and for the intraocular pressure to still be above the desired level; vitreous volume reduction requires longer time than reduction of anterior chamber pressure.[38]

Therefore, the careful surgeon or anesthesia provider watches both orbital and intraocular pressure in order to reduce vitreous volume for optimal surgical conditions.

When device pressure in the range of 20 to 25 mmHg is applied over the globe, the device can be used before the eye is anesthetized to reduce pre-block intraocular pressure.

This causes no problems, except inconvenience; higher pressures cause discomfort and could induce the oculocardiac reflex.

This pre-block reduction decreases intraocular pressure to below normal so that after five minutes of decompression, one can inject anesthetic and expect intraocular pressure not to rise as high as if the device had not been applied.[44] This can be done prophylactically for persons with glaucoma in whom there is concern that the injection behind the eye may elevate intraocular pressure beyond that patient's medical threshold. For such patients injection volume should be divided among several smaller injections. Application of 20 to 25 mmHg pressure before the block is not uncomfortable, and the author has not seen any EKG changes with it.

The biggest advantage of the oculocompression device is that it allows repeated injections in the orbit to establish total orbital akinesia and anesthesia, and provides a controlled intraocular pressure and volume equal to or less than that prior to injection.

Most cataract surgeons would like the vitreous volume less than normal and the orbital volume as low as possible so that no fluid pressure exists against the speculum applied to the globe, especially in a deep set eye. Most vitreoretinal surgeons are pleased with an increase in orbital volume that helps to bring the globe up for easier access to the muscles and the posterior aspect of the globe.

Oculocompression can be used to aid the oculoplastic surgeon; after injections are made in the lid, the device can be put in place, and within five minutes, usually all the puffiness from anesthetic injection in the lid will disappear, leaving the creases as they were and the anatomic relationships undisturbed by the additional volume of fluid.

Hamilton used the Super Pinky® for many years and has recently switched to the Honan balloon®. Hustead used the Honan balloon® for many years then switched to a home-made bulb syringe with very low wall tension. The indentation in the end of the bulb syringe allows application without putting as much pressure on the cornea as with most other compression devices whose surfaces are planar or convex (refer to Figure 3.25). The concavity of the syringe helps keep the lids closed.

Thus oculocompression has significantly benefitted the anesthesia provider allowing larger volumes of anesthetic and augmentation without increasing orbital volume prior to cataract surgery. Judicious use can allow augmentation and optimal increase in orbital volume, if that is desired by the retinal surgeon.

It is interesting to speculate how orbital decompression devices function. Otto has shown that whenever volume is injected in the orbit or pressure applied against the lids there is a rapid flow of fluid out of the orbit and a slow return to its original pressure.[45] Communication of the orbital veins with extraorbital veins may play a significant role in the process.

Current Techniques in Ophthalmic Anesthesia for Cataract or Vitreous Surgery

Those ophthalmologists who have made contributions in the literature by suggesting changes in anesthetic technique for cataract surgery were encouraged to submit a brief synopsis of their current techniques. The chapter authors' comments appear as "Editors' Comment."

This section is divided into two categories: Injection Anesthesia and Topical Anesthesia. Contributions are arranged in alphabetical order.

INJECTION ANESTHESIA

LEROY B. BLOOMBERG, MD, FACS, FICS
Bloomberg Eye Center, Newark, Ohio

"Bloomberg Anterior Periocular Anesthesia Technique (Orbital Epidural Anesthesia)"

For many years it has been traditional to use retrobulbar anesthesia when performing eye surgery. This technique has been described as early as 1884 by Knapp.[8] The most common technique used today is that which has been described by Atkinson. While complications of retrobulbar anesthesia are few, they can be quite serious. These complications include: retrobulbar hemorrhage, respiratory depression, intradural or subarachnoid injection, optic nerve damage and perforation of the eye. In hopes of eliminating serious complications, many surgeons have begun to use periocular anesthesia.

Retrobulbar anesthesia depends on a small volume (2 to 4 cc) of anesthesia injected into the muscle cone directly behind the eye (Figure 3.2). To do this, a long needle (1 1/4 to 1 1/2″) is used. The patient is typically advised to look superior nasally while the needle is placed along the outer third of the lower lid. Once the needle penetrates the skin about 1 cm, it is directed upward and nasally into the muscle cone. This also places the needle close to the posterior portion of the eye and near the optic nerve. Two to 4 cc of anesthetic is injected at this point. Because the needle is directed upward and inward, there is a chance, especially in long myopic eyes, that it could penetrate the globe (Figure 3.3).

Another possibly serious complication is optic nerve damage. Optic nerve damage can occur if too much anesthetic is injected in the retrobulbar space causing compression of the optic nerve. This could also occur if the needle penetrates the optic nerve sheath allowing the anesthetic to be injected directly along the optic nerve sheath (Figure 3.4). The latter would cause direct compression of the optic nerve. Another mechanism of optic nerve damage could occur if the needle is placed directly into the optic nerve. Compression of the optic nerve could result in central retinal vein occlusion and either of these complications could result in optic nerve atrophy and total blindness.[47-49] Injecting anesthetic into the optic nerve sheath could allow the anesthetic to enter the subarachnoid or subdural space, resulting in respiratory depression and even transient contralateral blindness as well as mid-brain anesthesia. To avoid many of these complications, it has been suggested that a dull needle be used, but this has not eliminated the problem.

Since 1983, I have been using periocular anesthesia,[34,46] hoping to eliminate some of these serious complications. Variations of this technique have been used by Davis, Weiss, Kelman, Pannu and many others.[50] My periocular anesthesia technique utilizes a shorter 27 gauge needle, 3/4 to 1″ long. The needle is deliberately directed away from the eye and the anesthetic is deliberately injected outside the muscle cone (Figure 3.5). For this technique to be successful, a much larger volume (8 to 10 cc) is required. Because the anesthetic must disperse around the orbit, the surgeon must allow 12 to 20 minutes for it to take effect.

Technique

Before administering anterior periocular anesthesia, the anesthetist injects small doses of sublimaze (Fentanyl) or midazolam intravenously. The sedation is titrated

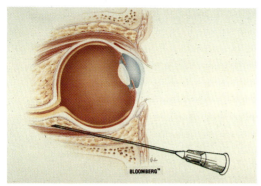

Figure 3.2. Retrobulbar anesthesia requires that the anesthetic is injected into the muscle cone directly behind the eye.

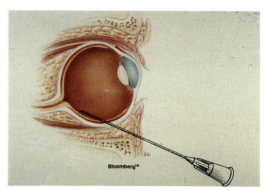

Figure 3.3. A potential complication of retrobulbar anesthesia is globe penetration.

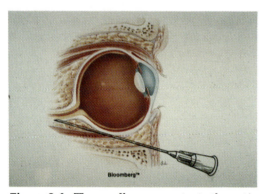

Figure 3.4. The needle can penetrate the optic nerve sheath allowing the anesthetic to be injected directly along the optic nerve sheath with the use of retrobulbar anesthesia.

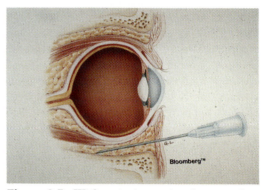

Figure 3.5. With anterior periocular anesthesia, the needle is deliberately directed away from the eye and the anesthetic is deliberately injected outside the muscle cone.

slowly until the patient is relaxed. The patient is monitored and vital signs are recorded.

Eight to 10 cc of the mixture is drawn up after warming it to increase patient comfort. The anesthesia mixture is a combination of one vial (150 cc) of hyaluronidase (Wydase), 15 cc of 0.75% bupivacaine (Marcaine), and 15 cc of 2% carbocaine. Sodium bicarbonate (0.2 cc) is added to each 10 cc of the mixture. A 3/4" 27 gauge needle is placed inferior temporally at the junction of the outer one-third and inner two-thirds of the lower lid (Figure 3.6). The needle is directed toward the floor of the orbit, away from the eye. A 3/4" needle is advanced to the hub. A 1" needle is advanced 3/4"; not to the hub. The anesthetic is slowly injected until the entire 8 to 10 cc have been injected or the orbit becomes full.

After the needle is withdrawn, the lids are taped closed and a Honan pressure cuff is placed over the eye with the pressure set at 30 to 40 mmHg. Approximately *12 to 20 minutes* is required for the anesthetic to disperse around the orbit and become totally effective, so periocular anesthesia should be administered at least 20 minutes before beginning surgery. During this time, the pressure gauge should be checked. As the

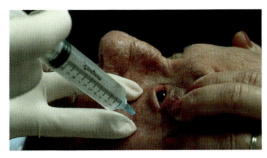

Figure 3.6. A 3/4" 27 gauge needle is placed inferior temporally at the junction of the outer one-third and inner two-thirds of the lower lid.

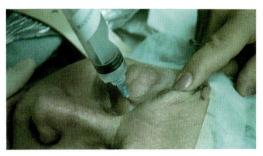

Figure 3.7. Additional anesthesia can be administered superior nasally.

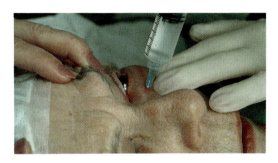

Figure 3.8. Additional anesthesia can also be administered inferior nasally or superior temporally depending on which muscle is not effectively blocked.

anesthetic disperses, the eye will soften and it may be necessary to reset the pressure on the Honan cuff to 30 to 40 mmHg.

In a small percentage of cases it may be necessary to use supplemental anesthesia if the first injection is not completely effective. Additional anesthesia can be administered superior nasally, inferior nasally or superior temporally depending on which muscle is not effectively blocked (Figures 3.7, 3.8).

Summary

Periocular anesthesia is a safe and effective method for ocular anesthesia and akinesia. It can be used by ophthalmic surgeons, anesthesiologists and nurse anesthetists with relative ease. Re-blocks may be necessary in 30 to 50% of cases when learning the technique, but once the technique is mastered, this rate drops to less than 10%. My experience has shown that complete anesthesia may be obtained with only one periocular injection, but as with retrobulbar anesthesia, some slight movement is still possible.

Editors' Comment

If one plans to obtain akinesia of the globe with "periocular" technique, one should learn to make safe supplemental injections. Dr. Hustead visited Dr. Bloomberg in 1990 while a new preceptee was training. All blocks done by the preceptee needed infra-nasal and supra-nasal injections to produce akinesia. The 3/4" needles for the supplements were placed tangential to the equator, about 10° central toward the optical axis and about at the hind surface of the globe—thus far from the optic nerve but probably in the anterior oculomotor compartment.

DAVID B. DAVIS II, MD, FACS
MARK R. MANDEL, MD.
Medical Surgical Eye Center, Hayward, California

Modified from
"Peribular Anesthesia,
A Review of Techniques and Complications"

Drs. Davis and Mandel, with their publication of peribulbar anesthesia[28] in 1986, startled the ophthalmic world using an alternative term for injections of anesthetic blocks behind the eye—namely, "peribulbar anesthesia." In their original publication, a 35 to 38 mm Atkinson short beveled needle was placed deep in the orbit in the periorbital space in the infero-temporal and supero-nasal quadrants instead of in the muscle cone (Figure 3.9). The technique has since been modified to the use of a blunt, 23 or 25 gauge, 7/8" needle.

They currently use a mixture of two parts 0.75% bupivacaine and one part 1% lidocaine without epinephrine to which they add 0.1 to 0.25 ml of hyaluronidase in a 10 ml syringe.

The skin wheal is made according the author's diagram in the preferred locus (A) of Figure 3.10a and b. Figure 3.11 shows the needle site of injection just anterior to the equator and figure 3.12 is deposition just past the equator. The superficial injection of the mixture of BSS/lidocaine is given at the junction of the lateral 1/3 and medial 2/3 of the lower lid just above the inferior orbital rim using a 1/2" 27 gauge needle. A total of 2 ml is given. They go through that same site A to make their "peribulbar" injection.

A peribulbar needle (a blunt 23 or 25 gauge 7/8 BD or a 7/8" Thornton needle) is introduced at the same location as the skin injection (Figure 3.11) and 1 ml is deposited in the orbicularis before the needle is advanced just anterior to the equator of the globe where 2 or 3 ml are deposited. Then the needle is advanced past the equator (Figure 3.12), remaining outside the cone where an additional 4 to 7 ml of anesthetic is administered.

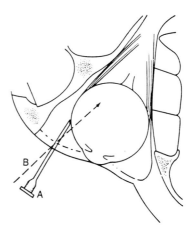

Figure 3.9. Superior view. (A) direction of peribulbar injection; (B) direction of retrobulbar injection.

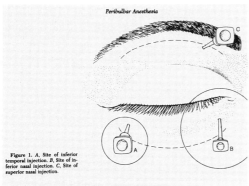

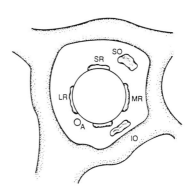

Figure 1. *A*, Site of inferior temporal injection. *B*, Site of inferior nasal injection. *C*, Site of superior nasal injection.

Figure 3.10a. (A) Site of injection; (B) & (C) Optional sites for injection.

Figure 3.10b. Location of peribulbar needle (A) at x-section of the globe near the equator.

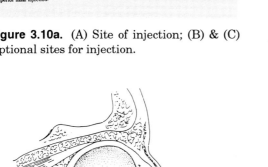

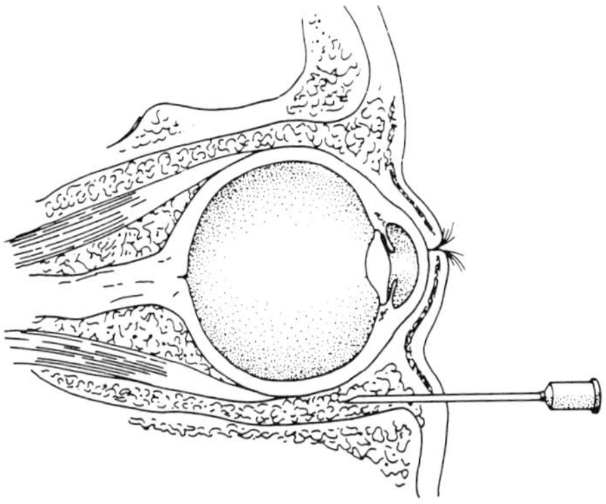

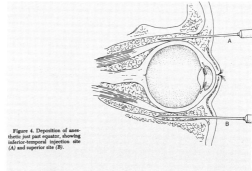

Figure 4. Deposition of anesthetic just past equator, showing inferior-temporal injection site (A) and superior site (B).

Figure 3.11. Deposition of anesthetic just anterior to the equator.

Figure 3.12. Deposition of anesthetic just past the equator, showing inferior-temporal injection site (A) and superior site (B).

The injection is given slowly, stopping when the superior lid fold disappears. A volume of 6 to 8 ml is usually injected.

Ten minutes following the block ocular motility is evaluated. If there is minor movement, the authors believe it will continue to lessen; however, if major motion exists at 10 minutes, then an additional injection is made through preferentially site B in their diagram at the junction of the medial 1/3 and lateral 2/3 of the lower lid at the inferior orbital rim. Several milliliters of anesthetic are injected slightly anterior to the equator and several are injected slightly posterior to the equator. The authors note that usually some residual ocular movement remains, but has not interfered with surgery.

Davis and Mandel believe that following the peribulbar injection, if slight proptosis and bulging of the supero-nasal lid fold are observed proper placement of anesthetic can almost be assured and that almost complete akinesia and anesthesia will result from a single injection. Immediately following injection, a Super Pinky® is placed for 15 to 30 minutes with three 4x4 gauze pads separating the Super Pinky® from the lid.

Dr. Davis has initiated an extensive reporting program to validate the safety of peribulbar anesthesia.[50]

Editors' Comment

Orbital block techniques involving injections outside the muscle cone into the periorbital space referred to by Davis and Mandel as "posterior peribulbar" anesthesia in 1986 were advocated by them to avoid the optic nerve and conal structures. Their original publication placed the injection site in almost the same place advocated by Braun[34b] in 1918, Labat[52] in 1926, and Pitkin[53a] in 1946—and for the same reason—to be completely away from the optic nerve and ophthalmic artery. The failure of orbital techniques to provide reliable anesthesia for enucleation or akinesia for cataract surgery led to their abandonment in the 1940s.

The supero-nasal orbital block had been credited with a number of cases of blindness before 1948;[53b] it was recommended that needles not be placed posterior to the posterior ethmoidal foramen or 20 mm past the fronto-nasal suture.

Posterior periorbital techniques suffered from the lack of reliability due to the varying shape of the orbit and varying shape of the orbital fissures used as landmarks when the needle was walked along the orbit. The object was to avoid entering the cone at the apex where damage to structures could occur. A small volume of 1 to 2 ml was injected at each site.

"Posterior peribulbar" anesthesia omitted the use of bony landmarks and needle placed points deep in the orbit where 4 ml of anesthetic was injected in both an infero-temporal and supero-nasal site. Akinesia and anesthesia of the globe and orbicularis were reliable.

Complications (apnea, optic nerve trauma, and perforation) reported by others learning the technique of "posterior peribulbar" block led Davis to advocate shorter needles for more anterior placement of the anesthetic. Davis and Mandel changed the name of the block to "anterior peribulbar" in 1990. Depth to which needles are inserted and the direction needles take to avoid perforation still make the technique a problem for some.

ANIBAL GALINDO, MD, PhD
Cedars Medical Center, Coral Gables, Florida

Retro-Peribulbar Anesthesia

The development and refinement of drugs and techniques have contributed to a widespread use of regional anesthesia for ophthalmic surgery. With a greater range of choices, the complications and side effects concurrent with its use become apparent. An effort should be made to understand the underlying anatomic and pharmacologic factors that contribute to these complications and the technical corrections necessary to turn retro-peribulbar anesthesia into a safe and complication-free technique.

Technical Considerations

In performing ophthalmic anesthesia through retro-peribulbar injections, consideration for a safe technique should address the following complications:

1. Intraoptic nerve injection, resulting in subarachnoid injection, optic nerve damage, and obstruction thrombosis of central vessels of the retina.
2. Laceration of the ophthalmic artery and, therefore, retrobulbar hemorrhage or intra-arterial injection.
3. Perforation of the globe.
4. Persistent diplopia or palpebral ptosis.
5. High peribulbar pressure.

Complications 1 through 3 can be traced to the sharp needle tips presently used and could be eliminated by using truly blunt needles, such as the pinlike needle introduced to ophthalmic anesthesia following its experimental success in eliminating the damage to the peripheral nerves otherwise inflicted by ordinary cutting needles.

In addition to the configuration of the tip, needles used for retro-peribulbar anesthesia should not be longer than 31 mm, taking into consideration that the depth of the bony orbit is only 40 mm.

Persistent diplopia and palpebral ptosis are caused by direct toxicity of the local anesthetic on the extraocular muscles. This toxicity should be reduced by using lower concentrations of these drugs, especially bupivacaine (less than 0.5%) and etidocaine (less than 1%). High periocular pressure, especially retrobulbar, may cause occlusion of retinal vessels with temporary or permanent blindness. There are two causes for this pressure rise during retrobulbar injections: (1) hemorrhage and (2) rapid increase in volume within a tight muscle cone compartment. Slow injections using noncutting needles and careful observation should eliminate this complication.

Following the standard principles of anesthesia care, patients undergoing retro-peribulbar anesthesia should be monitored with continuous ECG, blood pressure, and peripheral oxygen saturation. The use of drugs for sedation should be restricted to only those patients in whom gentle reassurance and persuasion fail to calm apprehension. An intravenous line should be started in all patients to ensure rapid administration of any emergency medications that may be required.

Technique

Based on the previously discussed technical considerations, the anatomic characteristics of the orbit and the eye, and the pharmacology of presently available local anesthetics, a technique for retro-peribulbar anesthesia has been developed by the author.

Two injections and two different drugs at each site are used: an inferior retrobulbar (mostly for motor blockade) and a superior retro-peribulbar (mostly for sensory anesthesia).

For the inferior retrobulbar injections, the goal is to obtain a profound and rapid anesthesia of most motor nerves. This can be achieved with 3 to 4 ml of mepivacaine 2% (Carbocaine) buffered to a pH of 7.2 and with the addition of hyaluronidase. (To a vial of 20 ml of Carbocaine 2%, add 150 units of hyaluronidase and 2 ml of sodium bicarbonate 8.4%.)

With the superior retro-peribulbar injections, the goal is to obtain long lasting sensory anesthesia and a blockade of terminal branches of three motor nerves (cranial nerves VII, III, VI, and IV). This can be obtained by injecting 3 to 4 ml of bupivacaine 0.5% or less (Marcaine, Sensorcaine) buffered to pH 7.0 and with hyaluronidase (to a vial of 20 ml, add 150 units of hyaluronidase and 0.2 ml of sodium bicarbonate 8.4%). The combination of these two sites of injection and two different anesthetic solutions should provide akinesia with complete surgical anesthesia in less than 10 minutes.

The two injections should be safe, with minimal discomfort for the patient and of simple execution. The site of penetration on the skin is infiltrated with local anesthetic through a 30 gauge needle, preferably with the same mepivacaine 2%, which is later used for the inferior retrobulbar approach. The anesthetic solutions are delivered by attaching a short (3 to 6 inches) extension tube between the syringe and the needle. The needle to perform the retro-peribulbar injections should not have a cutting tip but a pin-like tip with side port (Pinpoint). It should be 25 or 27 gauge, 31 mm long, straight or, preferably with a 135-degree angle that shortens the length to 28 mm from the hub to the tip. Because this needle does not cut tissues but separates them, the resistance to penetration is greater and the advance should be made with a firm push while palpating the space between the ocular globe and the orbit.

This special needle has been used for more than five years in several centers and in over 7000 retro-peribulbar injections without serious complications. As expected, the safer pin-like tip presents a technical inconvenience because penetration of the skin and other tissues is obviously more difficult than with the cutting needle and may cause some pain. This inconvenience is reduced with local anesthetic infiltration at the site of penetration. This penetration should be firm and properly directed, and if the angled needle is used, it should follow the roof or the floor of the orbit, away from the ocular globe and then directed to an imaginary point 4 to 10 mm behind the eye.

The use of a pin-like needle is likely to eliminate one of the most serious complications in ophthalmic anesthesia, such as the penetration of the optic nerve, that may result in subarachnoid injection of the local anesthetic, optic nerve palsy, and/or thrombosis of the retinal vessels. Penetration of the optic nerve is very unlikely using a pin-like type of needle because the nerve will be displaced before it could be penetrated. Penetration of the eye globe, the other serious complications of retro-as well as peribulbar blocks, is also unlikely to occur with the pin-like tip needle since the high resistance of the sclera to this needle rotates the ocular globe when forced against it, alerting the operator to the dangers of the needle direction and the impending penetration of the globe, a warning non-existant with the sharp needles. Advancing the needle through the skin and subcutaneous tissue is, as expected, more difficult with the pin-like tip than with the sharp needles (Atkinson and ordinary disposable).

Editors' Comment

Galindo has been in the forefront of regional anesthesia for many years as an advocate of the pinpoint needle for regional anesthesia to avoid intravascular or intraneural injection. He has applied this regional anesthesia needle and his knowledge of orbital anatomy to reducing the complications of retrobulbar block anesthesia in his hospital. He bends the 25 or 27 gauge 1.25″ needles, then places one in the infero-temporal and one in the supero-nasal quadrant. He very slowly injects local anesthetic through these needles. The needles have a pin-point opening which is non-cutting and a side port to allow the anesthetic to leave 3 mm behind the point of the needle (Figure 3.1).

These needles require special technique and special training. As the port passes through minor septa there is elastic recoil of the septa which can catch elastic tissue in septa. This causes the eye to move—a sign that indicates the needle is in thick septa, or Tenon's—an absolute rule to withdraw the needle.

Dr. Galindo believes the non-cutting point of the needle has specific benefit in preventing inadvertent perforation of the globe. Research along this line is being conducted by Dr. Galindo and the staff of Bascom/Palmer Eye Institute in Miami and has produced the data for Table 3.1.

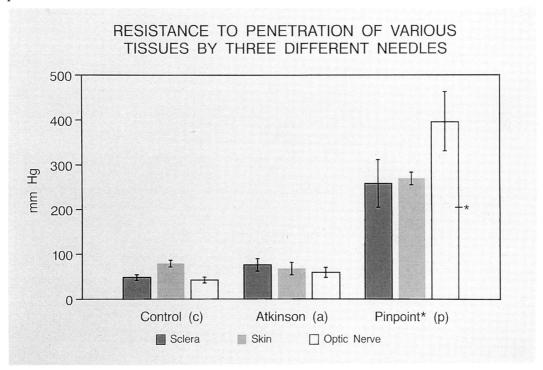

Table 3.1. Comparison of the grams of force needed to perforate the skin, and the sclera. On the left, a 25 gauge regular sharp Monoject® needle; in the center, with a 25 gauge Atkinson disposable needle, and on the right with the 25 gauge Pinpoint needle. Notice in all cases it takes about the same grams of force to penetrate the skin that it takes to penetrate the sclera with each of the needles and that the force required of a 25 gauge sharp needle is approximately the same as with an Atkinson needle.

JAMES P. GILLS, MD
TOM LOYD, PA
St. Luke's Cataract & Laser Institute, Tarpon Springs, Florida

Anesthesia for Ophthalmic Surgery

Procedure

The patient is positioned comfortably lying back at a height that is comfortable for the anesthetist. An examining chair is excellent for this because it has an adjustable headrest, the anesthetist can get close to the patient to line up landmarks for the injection and also watch the eye and needle closely without getting a backache. The patient is given a fixation point on the ceiling to keep the eye in the primary gaze, or preferably slightly upward. Medial gaze is avoided. If the patient has strabismus, the head or chair or both is rotated to attain the proper gaze in order to avoid rotating the optic nerve toward the injection site.

One drop of painless proparacaine (solution preparation below) is instilled in the lower lid and the eye is closed. After a few seconds, one drop of full strength proparacaine is instilled in the lower lid and the eye is closed again for a few seconds. The patient is instructed to watch the fixation object and is allowed to blink as needed. Lidocaine 1% with epinephrine 1.5 ml, in a 3 ml syringe with a 27 gauge 1.25 inch needle (Monoject), is injected trans-conjunctivally to the level of the muscle cone, over a period of 20-30 seconds. This is given about 5 mm from the lateral canthus in the infero-lateral cul-de-sac.

After waiting a few seconds, the retrobulbar injection is given over a period of about one minute, passing through the anesthetized area. Again the patient's gaze is directed as before. Marcaine 0.75% with epinephrine 5 ml is given in the retrobulbar space. The needle is directed close to the globe in a line lateral to the lateral limbal margin. It is important to enter the muscle cone and this is usually confirmed by ballooning of the conjunctiva during injection. A 25 gauge 1.25 inch needle (Monoject) is used and usually inserted the full length. After the injection the eye is closed and no pressure is applied *unless there is evidence of retrobulbar hemorrhage.*

After two minutes, the Super Pinky® is applied to the eye over a 2 X 2 gauze square for two minutes to spread the medicine. The eye muscle movements are evaluated and one of the following courses is taken.

1. If there is slight movement in several muscles, a repeat retrobulbar injection of 3 to 5 ml of carbocaine 2% is given. This works rapidly and is rechecked after one minute with the Super Pinky®.

2. If there is movement of the medial rectus with or without movement of the superior rectus, a medial peri-conal injection of 2-4 ml carbocaine 2% is given, and the eye rechecked after one minute with the Super Pinky®.

3. If there is movement of the superior rectus only, a lateral superior peri-conal or medial superior peri-conal injection of 2-4 ml carbocaine 2% is given, and the eye is rechecked after one minute compression with the Super Pinky®.

Full strength marcaine 0.75% should not be used for medial or superior peri-conal injections due to possible toxic effects on muscles with resultant upper lid ptosis or fibrosis of the medial rectus.

After checking to ensure total akinesia, a surgical bonnet is placed on the patient's head, and the Super Pinky® is placed over the closed operative eye over a 2 X 2 gauze square. The pressure and position of the ball is adjusted to allow about 30 mmHg pressure on the eye.

The patient is allowed to be ambulatory as needed to prepare for surgery. The Super Pinky® is left on 20 to 60 minutes to lower the pressure in the eye, and should not be used prior to the block due to the risk of vaso-vagal response.

Preparing Your Medications

Painless Eye Drop

Take the plunger out of a 3 ml syringe and drop in 0.25 ml of proparacaine. Add 1.5 ml BSS and several drops of sodium bicarbonate 8.4% (check the pH with pH paper and adjust the amount of sodium bicarbonate added to reach a pH of 7.4), replace plunger, inject into an empty dropper bottle, and label. The solution is stable for two days. This is very useful in other areas of the clinic. An alternative is to add 0.5 ml proparacaine to a 15 ml bottle of artificial tears.

Pre-retrobulbar: To a 50 ml multidose bottle of lidocaine 1% with epinephrine, add about 3.5 ml sodium bicarbonate 8.4% (available in a crash cart vial or 50 ml multidose bottle), add 0.25 ml (37.5 units) Wydase. Check the pH to attain the proper amount of bicarbonate to add. Lidocaine without epinephrine comes at a higher pH to begin with, and requires less bicarbonate addition.

Retrobulbar: To a 30 ml vial of 0.75% Marcaine with epinephrine add about 1 ml bicarb 8.4%. Check pH to attain pH of about 6.2-6.4, Marcaine comes out of solution at a pH of 6.8) add Wydase 0.15 ml (22 units).

Or to a 30 ml vial of 0.75% Marcaine without epinephrine add only the Wydase. (The pH is already about 6.2-6.5 from the manufacturer). Epinephrine may be added if you wish 0.15 ml of 1:1,000.

Peri-conal: To a 50 ml bottle of carbocaine 2% add 3.5 ml of bicarb 8.4%, and 0.25 ml Wydase (37.5 units). This can also be used for a safe, comfortable, rapid, retrobulbar, which will last only one to two hours.

Summary

We have found some basic guidelines of importance:

1. Have the patient look in the primary gaze or slightly upward, but not nasally, as this will rotate the optic nerve toward the injection site.
2. Inject transconjunctivally in the infero-lateral cul-de-sac between the inferior rectus and lateral rectus along a path lateral to the extended limbal margin to keep well lateral to the optic nerve.
3. Keep close to the globe with the bevel toward the globe so the muscle cone can be entered with the least possible needle length. In this larger portion of the muscle cone, the structures are more spread out and less susceptible to damage.
4. Always check the axial length of the eye prior to injection.
5. During transconjunctival injection, if the sclera is touched, the eye will turn downward, replace the needle to avoid the globe. This only works with a transconjunctival injection. With a transcutaneous injection, the globe could be pierced with no motion evident, due to the sharper angle of approach.

6. We try to be flexible with the injections, doing whatever seems appropriate (such as injecting in selected periconal areas for particular muscle activity).

7. For newcomers to retrobulbar injections, or those with difficulty getting help in an emergency, it is advisable to give the retrobulbar in two or three small doses, waiting a few minutes between, with no pressure on the eye. This way there is less chance of sending a large bolus to the sub-arachnoid space, if the optic nerve sheath is pierced

Editors' Comment

The lateral cone technique of Gills and Loyd[26] was published in 1983 to call attention to lid akinesia, which occurred after infero-temporal injection in their technique of "retrobulbar block."

The 1983 article was important for other historical, anatomical, and pharmacologic reasons. It was the first U.S. published modification of retrobulbar technique to utilize the anatomical information from the CT scans reported by Unsold et al[54].

Gills and Loyd modified their retrobulbar block technique several years before publishing it. They did so to prevent "Marcaine®" apnea which had occurred in several patients which they assumed came from injection in the optic nerve sheath by the mechanism which Unsold[54] described. Two efforts where thus made to keep the optic nerve away from the retrobulbar needle: (1) to avoid the supero-nasal position, and (2) to purposely direct the needle into the lateral cone away from the optic nerve. The price paid for avoiding the central cone was paresis of the extraocular muscles rather than akinesia from the primary injection, so repeat injection at five minutes was recommended to accomplish total akinesia, which was achieved in 99.5% of cases.

The technique also decreased the pain of eye blocks and avoided sedatives by the use of topical anesthesia, 27 gauge sharp needles, the transconjunctival approach, a preliminary injection of less painful 1% lidocaine to precede more painful bupivacaine, and slow timed injection of local anesthetic. Finally, the report verified prolonged post-operative analgesia as a uniform feature of large volume blocks, when a "perfect block" was established before surgery.

This technique has now been used in over 50,000 patients by Gills and staff with no known damage to the optic nerve and no cases of perforation of the globe. A single case of apnea occurred when a new preceptee embarked on a solo block, but the patient recovered without sequelae and there have been none since.

Such a safety record is possible only because of the conscientious nature in which Tom Loyd has taught those who work with him to follow the principles of the block. The block was modified[27] only slightly since its inception to include pH adjustment of anesthetic solution; a medial compartment block through the medial canthus for patients in whom that compartment requires additional anesthetic instead of the five minute repeat injection in the lateral cone.

Hustead has watched Tom Loyd and his colleagues do many blocks and is pleased to report that they put needles where the illustrations of 1983 depict (see Figure 3.13, 3.14) with two exceptions. The first block is usually done with the needle point as depicted and the hub more anterior to the inferior orbital rim; whereas, the second injection is usually done with the hub as depicted and the needle point 4 to 5 mm further posterior. There is an artists' perspective error in Figure 3.14; the globe is oversized to draw attention to the equator and the path of the needle.

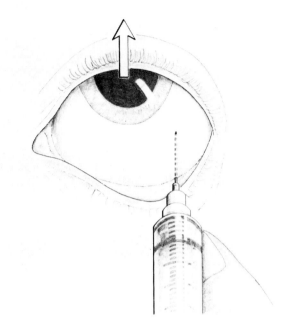

Figure 3.13. The retrobulbar injection is directed in line with the lateral limbal margin with the eye looking upward but nasally.

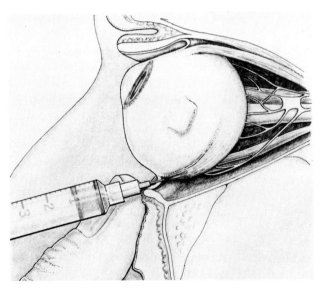

Figure 3.14. Transconjunctival injection is tangential to the globe. The slightest scleral contact will cause the eye to turn downward. Puncture of the globe is less likely than with a transcutaneous injection.

W. SANDERSON GRIZZARD, MD
Family Medical Arts Center, Tampa, Florida

Regional Ophthalmic Anesthesia

When using regional anesthesia for retinal surgery, it is necessary to consider the alternatives and to ensure that patients are selected carefully. The great majority of patients undergoing cataract surgery can be done under local anesthesia; the same is not true for retinal and vitreous surgery.

Two additional factors that make the use of regional anesthesia more difficult are that the procedures last much longer and that there is greater manipulation of the muscles and periocular tissue. It is much easier to do a vitrectomy under local anesthesia than to perform a scleral buckling under local.

It is also important to consider not only patient variables, such as cooperation and health, but also the operating environment. In hospitals which are familiar with my technique, I am more comfortable using local anesthesia. In unfamilar surroundings or at night, when the operating room personnel may be unfamiliar with the surgical techniques, general anesthesia is advised.

Anesthetic Mixture

I use a 1/1 or 2/1 mixture of 0.75% Marcaine and 4% Xylocaine. For surgery of short duration, such as removal of a plaque or tap for endophthalmitis, 2% Xylocaine buffered with bicarbonate is used.

My injection is started with a 27 gauge 1 1/4" sharp pointed disposable needle. A sharp needle is used because I believe that an Atkinson style blunt needle offers no additional safety but increases the pain and need for perioperative sedation.

The block is begun with a retrobulbar injection using 3 to 4 ml of anesthetic with the eye in primary gaze. The needle is passed posteriorly until it passes the equator of the eye and then direct it toward a hypothetical position approximately .5 cm behind the macula. I formerly placed the needle to its maximum depth, but following the recommendations of Dr. Bloomberg,[30] it is evident that better anesthesia is obtained with the needle at approximately 3/4 to 1 inch depth. The needle is retracted and redirected straight posteriorly to approximately 1 to 1 1/4 depth. The needle is retracted another cc is injected under the skin in the method suggested by Kimbrough[74] for lid akinesia. At this point I withdraw the needle and place pressure on the eye.

Then 3 cc are injected superonasally using a 1/2 inch needle through the caruncle directing the needle superiorly as described by Hustead and Hamilton. This latter technique gives excellent ocular anesthesia for vitrectomy, however, I still have difficulty getting good anesthesia along the superior rectus muscle and many of my patients complain of pain when a suture is placed under the superior rectus muscle.

If there is superior pain I inject superotemporally using the 27 gauge 1 1/4 inch needle injecting slightly temporal to the supero-orbital notch being very careful to keep the needle tip along the superior orbital wall to avoid penetrating the eye. The eye is closest to the orbit superiorly and a needle directed straight posteriorly can penetrate the globe due to the overhang of the superior orbital rim. I sometimes proceed with a Van Lint block. Often this is unnecessary but it can greatly facilitate the manipulation of the eye in an uncooperative patient. A gauze pad is used to apply pressure to the eye for approximately five minutes. It is rare not to have adequate anesthesia and akinesia with this type of block.

After beginning surgery, if there is pain in a local area, I inject locally along the rectus muscle using 2% Xylocaine. I also occaisionally use a blunt cannula and irrigate the Tenon's tissue behind the eye in four quadrants for added infiltration of anesthesia.

Combined Technique

An excellent alternative to either straight local or straight general anesthesia is to use a combined technique. Following intubation and anesthetic induction, a reteobulbar injection can be given with Marcaine. Because anesthesia is obtained by the block the patient can be maintained under a lighter level of anesthesia, and generally without narcotics. This allows quick recovery and minimal postoperative nausea. The additional postoperative analgesia is very useful in the initial postoperative period.

Editors' Comments

Dr. Grizzard very cogently describes the anatomic considerations for doing the cone injection block that he does and has allowed us to reproduce several of his drawings in this book.[55]

Dr. Grizzard has been a main force in using CT scans in Unsold's paper to avoid the supero-nasal position. However, Dr. Grizzard adopted this technique before CT scans had verified the mobility of the optic nerve. During his retinal fellowship an optic nerve was damaged by the "Atkinson" technique which led to intensive study of the course of the optic nerve and modifications of retrobulbar technique to minimize that risk. Dr. Grizzard's devotion to anterior placement of needles in the retrobulbar space puts him in the minority of retinal surgeons, many of whom use some modification of Gifford-type blocks to produce profound akinesia and anesthesia of long-lasting duration for vitreoretinal surgery.

ROBERT C. HAMILTON, MB, BCh
Calgary, Alberta, CANADA

Gimbel Eye Centre Technique of Ocular Regional Anesthesia

The author has provided ocular regional anesthesia for 28,000 cataract extraction and intraocular lens implantation procedures since the Gimbel Eye Surgical Centre opened in January 1984. In 1988 a report on the management of the first 12,000 anesthesias was published.[56] Five distinct techniques of injection were studied following which it was determined that a method incorporating an initial retrobulbar (intracone) injection, with or without peribulbar (pericone) supplementation, was most suited to the rapid turnover practice. Future dependence on solely peribulbar anesthesia was abandoned because of the time consuming higher supplementation requirement and need for larger intraorbital injectate volume. Definitive seventh nerve blocking is not used as sufficient spread to orbicularis oculi muscle follows appropriate intraorbital injection placement, confirming the 1983 report of Gills and Loyd[26] and the 1986 evaluation by Martin et al.[57]

The method described below uses fine sharp cutting disposable needles which, although controversial,[58] have been endorsed by this author[56] and by Grizzard et al.[59] Although a commonly held belief among ophthalmologists, it is not true that it is more difficult to penetrate the globe, the optic nerve sheath or blood vessels with a blunt needle.[59] Because disposable cutting needles produce minimal tissue distortion, little or no pain results. Any needle advanced within the confines of the orbit has the potential of serious complication;[28] therefore it behooves any serious practitioner of ophthalmic regional anesthesia to know well the anatomy of the orbit and its contents, pharmacology of the local anesthetics and ophthalmologic medications, and physiology of the eye.[60] The principal complications of ocular regional anesthesia are globe penetration, orbital bleeding, brainstem anesthesia and myotoxicity. There is a need for residency programs to include more than a perfunctory exposure to orbital anesthesia.

Pertinent Anatomy and Applied Anatomy

In Figure 3.15 the outline of the globe is superimposed on a template of the orbit rim. The rim has a basic, albeit lop-sided, quadrilateral shape. The space available for needle access to the globe equator and to deeper orbit structures, between the globe and the orbit rim, is greatest at the inferotemporal quadrant (arrow, Figure 3.15); this area is also suitable because it is relatively avascular.

For needle access to the intracone compartment, the inferotemporal quadrant is again the route of choice because the lateral orbit rim is set back in line with the globe equator (Figure 3.16).

Figure 3.16 also demonstrates that the orbit, in sagittal section, is C-shaped rather than U-shaped with the greater overhang superiorly. The orbit floor (inferior orbit wall) rises at an angle of 10 degrees from front to back (Figure 3.17). In order to avoid trauma to the inferior oblique muscle, or its motor nerve, an inferotemporal needle placement should be lateral to the sagittal plane of the lateral limbus. Figure 3.18 shows the path of

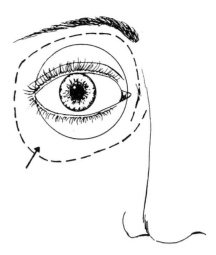

Figure 3.15. The outline of the globe is super-imposed on a template of the orbit rim.

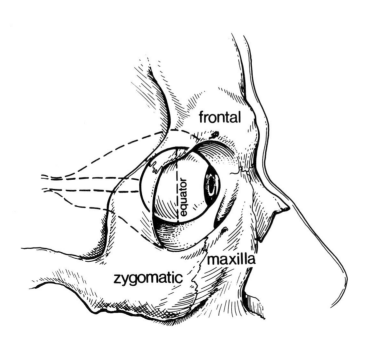

Figure 3.16. The lateral orbit rim is set back in line with the globe equator. The orbit, in sagittal section, is C-shaped rather than U-shaped with greater overhang superiorly. (Permission from W. Sanderson Grizzard, MD)

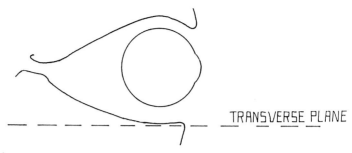

TRANSVERSE PLANE

Figure 3.17. The orbit floor (inferior orbit wall) rises at an angle of 10 degrees from front to back.

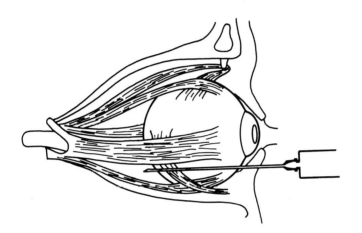

Figure 3.18. The path of a needle appropriately placed just inferior to the lower border of the lateral rectus muscle and well clear of the inferior oblique near its insertion into the globe. (Permission from H.S. Wang, MD and J Cataract Refract Surg)

a needle appropriately placed (just inferior to the lower border of the lateral rectus muscle and well clear of the inferior oblique near its insertion into the globe).

The trochlear nerve, motor supply to the superior oblique muscle, is the only oculomotor nerve whose path is outside the rectus muscle cone. Unlike the other five extraocular muscles, its motor supply enters the muscle on its orbital, not its conal surface. For these two reasons (both resulting in greater distance for injectate to spread) there is frequent retention of torque movement caused by persisting superior oblique activity following intracone anesthesia injection.

Needle Preparation

Two needles are used: one 30 gauge sharp disposable 12 mm and one 27 gauge sharp disposable 31 mm. The 27 gauge needle is bent to an angle of 10 degrees half way along its length by inserting inside a sterile 18 gauge needle. The bevel of the 27 needle should be in the concavity of the bend (Figure 3.19). The needle hub is marked with an indelible fibreglass pen to indicate the location of the bevel of the needle and the orientation of its angled distal half. The final needle tip position in the intracone compartment is 5.0 to 7.0

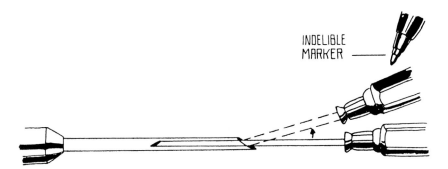

INDELIBLE
MARKER

Figure 3.19. The 27 gauge needle is bent to an angle of 10 degrees half way along its length by inserting a sterile 18 gauge needle. The bevel of the 27 needle should be in the concavity of the bend. The needle hub is marked with an indelible fiberglass pen to indicate the location of the bevel of the needle and the orientation of its angled distal half.

mm posterior to the posterior pole of the globe, having safely negotiated a track close to the orbit floor in the inferotemporal quadrant until past the globe equator. The end position of the needle tip will be at a depth of 25 to 31 mm[61] from the inferior orbit rim in the sagittal plane of the lateral limbus (see arrow, Figure 3.20) and with the globe lying in the concavity of the needle. Figure 3.20 is the view of the final needle position as seen from above: Figure 3.21 is the lateral view.

Anesthesia Mixture Preparation

The standard anesthesia mixture used for cataract extraction and intraocular lens implantation cases consists of 2.0% mepivacaine without preservative to which are added hyaluronidase (to 7.5 turbidity units per mL) and epinephrine (to a concentration of 1:200,000). Mepivacaine has a longer duration of action than lidocaine. When longer operations are contemplated or for slower surgeons an agent longer acting than mepivacaine may be selected but made up with the same additives.

A separate solution called "painless local" is made up by adding 1.5 mL of the standard mixture to a 15 mL plastic bottle of Alcon's *Balanced Salt Solution.*™

Patient Preparation and Management

Patients have preoperative history and physical done by their family physician. Much emphasis is placed on preliminary patient education, verbally by clinic staff and by audiovisual aids; an informed patient is a calm one. On the day of surgery patients sign a consent form outlining potential surgical and anesthesia complications and walk to the block room. They recline in a motorized contoured dental chair for the block procedure. An adhesive label displaying their name and bilateral axial length measurements is applied to their clothing over the shoulder on the side to be blocked and a small red tag to the forehead on the side of the proposed surgery.

Following establishment of full block, patients walk to a holding area, from where they are taken (remaining ambulatory) to the operating room as required. The operating table is a modified dental chair. Dental chairs, because of the comfort engendered by their contoured form, are well accepted by our patient population. During anesthesia and

Figure 3.20. View of the final needle position as seen from above. The end position of the needle tip will be at a depth of 25 to 31 mm from the inferior orbit rim in the sagittal plane of the lateral limbus (see arrow) and with the globe lying in the concavity of the needle. (Modified, with permission from W. Sanderson Grizzard MD)

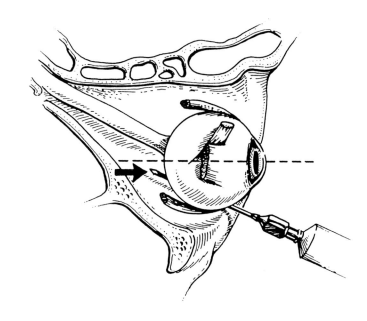

Figure 3.21. Side view of custom bent 27 gauge needle in final position in central intracone position.

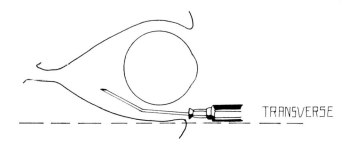

surgery non-invasive blood pressure, lead 1 EKG (wrist electrodes), pulse wave, and pulse oximetric monitoring are routine. Oxygen enrichment of humidified air under the drapes is adjusted according to the observed oxygen saturation.

Technique

Following topical anesthesia and appropriate ocular medications instilled into the conjunctival sac, the block procedures are performed.

The initial injection is of 1.0 mL "painless local" transconjunctivally and inferotemporally through the 30 gauge 12 mm needle, the tip entering just behind the inferior tarsal plate with the shaft of the needle arranged tangentially to the globe (Figure 3.22). The needle easily and painlessly (because of preliminary topical anesthesia drops) penetrates the conjunctiva, and deep to it the capsulo-palpebral fascia; 1.0 mL "painless local" is deposited at a depth of 1 cm from the conjunctiva (Figure 3.22). A one to two minutes wait establishes anesthesia along the track of the 27 gauge needle carrying

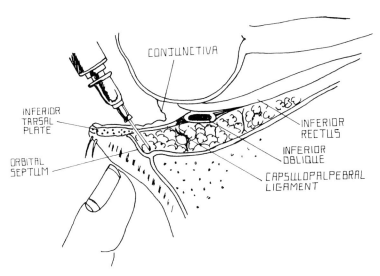

Figure 3.22. The initial injection is of 1.0 mL "painless local" transconjunctivally and inferotemporally through the 30 gauge 12-mm needle, the tip entering just behind the inferior tarsal plate with the shaft of the needle arranged tangentially to the globe. The needle easily and painlessly (because of preliminary topical anesthesia drops) penetrates the conjunctiva, and deep to it the capsulo-palpebral fascia; 1.0 mL "painless local" is deposited at a depth of 1 cm from the conjunctiva.

full-strength local anesthetic that follows. The rationale for the "painless local" injection is: to start the anesthesia process painlessly, to gain the confidence of the patient, to provide important feed-back to the practitioner about the "reactivity" and level of pain threshold of that individual.

The 27 gauge 31 mm specially bent disposable needle is mounted firmly on a 6.0 mL syringe filled with full-strength anesthesia mixture. The practitioner should palpate and become familiar with the location of the inferior orbit rim. The mid-sagittal plane of the globe should be visualized (Figure 3.20). With the patient's eye in primary gaze[54] the needle tip is inserted through conjunctiva, just posterior to the inferior tarsal plate and as far lateral as the given palpebral fissure will allow (inferior to the lower border of the lateral rectus muscle insertion into the globe as in Figure 3.18). The general direction of the needle and syringe assembly is medial to eventually attain a needle tip position in the sagittal plane of the lateral limbus (arrow, Figure 3.20) at a depth of 25 to 31 mm. The initial part of the needle placement entails advancing the leading half (15 mm) of the needle just over the inferior orbit rim and allowing it to rise slightly in keeping with the bony anatomy of the orbit floor (Figure 3.23) until the equator of the globe has been passed. In the second and final portion of the needle placement the second half of the needle has attained a position previously occupied by the leading half, i.e. parallel to the rising orbit floor (Figure 3.24). Following a test aspiration, injection is commenced to confirm absence of abnormal resistance; if any is suspected the needle tip should be relocated. While monitoring visually and digitally the increasing orbit volume and intracone pressure, (globe between finger and thumb of the non-injecting hand), 3.0 to 4.0 mL of the anesthesia mixture is injected s-l-o-w-l-y (two minutes).

Following a 10 minute period of orbit decompression with a Honan Balloon®[40] at a setting of 30 mmHg, the globe and periorbit are inspected in the usual manner in all four

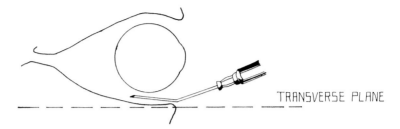

TRANSVERSE PLANE

Figure 3.23. The initial part of the needle insertion places the leading half (15 mm) of the needle just over the inferior orbit rim and allowing it to rise slightly in keeping with the bony anatomy of the orbit floor until the equator of the globe has been passed.

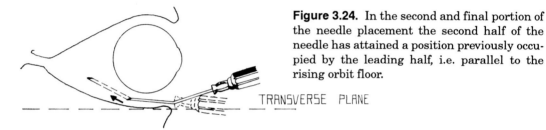

Figure 3.24. In the second and final portion of the needle placement the second half of the needle has attained a position previously occupied by the leading half, i.e. parallel to the rising orbit floor.

TRANSVERSE PLANE

quadrants. Many eyes will already be adequately anesthetized. Frequently persisting superior oblique activity or incomplete orbicularis oculi block will occur. A 2.0 to 4.0 mL injection through the 30 gauge 12 mm needle using the medial orbital pericone technique of Robert F. Hustead is effective. Occasionally repeat intracone blocking is required.

With complete akinesia, the Honan Balloon® is applied for a further 20 minute period at a pressure of 30 mmHg.

Editors' Comment

Dr. Hamilton changes his technique slightly about every 2,000 cases, so by the time this appears in print, he will have probably made some minor change.

ROBERT F. HUSTEAD, MD
Ochsner Eye Center, Wichita, Kansas

The Wichita Technique

Background

The author had the opportunity in 1974 to study a detailed scale model of the left orbit and dissect a number of orbits prior to doing eye blocks for patients. He has since anesthetized over 20,000 eyes and made over 50,000 injections into the orbit with a single retrobulbar hemorrhage, two perforations of the globe, and no cases of optic nerve injury or apnea. The circumstances of the injuries will be discussed because each occurred during departure from the technique which the author felt would be ideal based on analysis and orbital dissection.

The analysis suggested little tolerance in the orbit for errors in depth or angulation of needles. To prevent unwanted motion, patients were placed in light surgical anesthesia with sodium thiopental. An assistant maintained the airway and kept the head and eyelid in the desired position. Thiopental positioned the eyes straight ahead in the cadaveric position for anatomic reference (except in strabismus).

The 38 mm (1 1/2") 25 gauge Monoject® "standard needle" point was intended to go to the locus that the orbital model showed to be most void of structures—namely, in the space between the inferior and lateral rectus muscles approximately 5-8 mm from the hind surface of the eye 5 mm lateral to the optic nerve. The hub of the 38 mm needle was 5-8 mm anterior to the inferior orbital rim when the point was in position. The needle entered the skin over the inferior orbital rim at a point to take the needle midway between the lateral and inferior rectus muscles, then around the equator, and to follow a course parallel to the optic nerve lateral to the optical axis.

The shallow placement of the needle anterior to the muscle cone and parallel to the optic nerve was thought to prevent injury to the optic nerve and ophthalmic artery. Three ml of a 10 ml mixture of 2% lidocaine/0.25% tetracaine with 1:200,000 epinephrine and 150 I.U. of hyaluronidase was injected.

This "modified ciliary ganglion block" was preceded by a modified Van Lint block of the facial nerve to render the orbicularis inoperative and to test that the patient was in adequate depth of pentothal anesthesia for the eye block. After the retrobulbar injection, a supero-nasal injection was made just temporal to the supraorbital notch, hugging the superior roof, placing the needle point approximately 20 mm behind the plane of the iris where 2 ml of anesthetic was injected to block the trochlear and frontal nerves.

The block was checked at 10 minutes, and occasionally there was absence of anesthesia in the medial quadrant structures or poor akinesia in any quadrant. This was then supplemented by a second infero-temporal injection placed 5 mm further into the orbit.

This technique was used for 65 blocks without any injury. The next patient refused all sedatives or narcotics. The patient had a blood pressure of 180/90. The facial block was done first with moderate grimace, then a classical Atkinson block was planned using 2% lidocaine and having the patient look "up and in;" the 1-3/8" Atkinson point needle was placed through the infero-temporal quadrant with the globe supero-nasal as Atkinson described. The moment injection in the orbit started, the patient experienced extreme pain, and started a massive retrobulbar hemorrhage. Immediate pressure was applied.

The blood pressure was 230/120. The patient was rendered amnesic and cooperative by an intravenous injection of Pentothal®. Orbital pressure stopped the bleeding without canthotomy and surgery was postponed. Subsequent examination showed no visual loss from the hemorrhage. The patient's subsequent surgery was done six weeks later using general endotracheal anesthesia.

Following the retrobulbar hemorrhage, the author defined what would be done in order to avoid future retrobulbar hemorrhage. The cause of the hemorrhage was (1) an uncontrolled patient, (2) pre-existing systolic hypertension, and (3) the 23 gauge needle. Such conditions were controlled for all subsequent patients using a 27 ga. 1.25" (32 mm) needle and maintaining systolic pressure below 155 mmHg. No retrobulbar hemorrhage has occurred in over 50,000 injections behind the eye since adopting those criteria.

Approximately 2000 eye blocks before the two ocular perforations occurred. Both were in patients whose primary block produced little akinesia of the globe. Encouraged to use the safer 35 mm Atkinson needle so as to be able to place a needle closer to the globe and optic nerve to obtain better akinesia, the author had the patient look "up and in" to feel the "pop" of the intermuscular septum that would ensure that the needle was within the muscle cone rather than outside it.

The author was keenly aware of perforating the globe because he was looking for the feel of perforating the intermuscular septum and watched the globe move as the needle advanced; then with a bit of extra force to "penetrate the septum," the sclera injury was accomplished. This perforation occurred in a patient with a deep-set 28 mm elliptical myopic eye and a small orbital opening.

The author watched the vitreoretinal surgeon expose the wound of the injured eye and noticed that, contrary to description, there was no intermuscular septum in the area where the injury took place. Therefore the primary block was not unsatisfactory because of failure to penetrate an intermuscular septum; the patient had a long generous orbit which needed a large volume of anesthetic. The patient eventually lost sight after three vitrectomies.

The second scleral penetration occurred with a specially-dulled Atkinson needle, and led to the conclusion that a dull needle could not be relied upon to move the globe away from its point, especially if motion of the globe was detected during advancement of the needle.

The same year that these two injuries occurred, the author studied the Unsold[57] paper and its references to Koornneef's work, which ably demonstrated other areas in the orbit to make injections to augment akinesia when a shallow infero-temporal injection provided unsatisfactory akinesia. The author used four areas—the supero-temporal, the supero-nasal, the infero-nasal, or the medial pericone, depending upon what area needed to be supplemented. Gradually, the author convinced himself of the superiority of the medial canthal approach to the medial adipose tissue compartment and abandoned the supero-nasal and infero-nasal percutaneous sites even though no major bleeding had occurred from the use of those two sites in his hands. The medial site seemed to produce the needed supplementation in most patients, except for an occasional patient who had persistence of superior rectus or levator activity, and for those the author switched to a supero-temporal injection, eliminating the supero-nasal supplementary injection which he had used for many years. The supero-temporal technique is still used today when initial infero-temporal and medial pericone (with the needle directed 20° superiorly) fails to block the superior rectus.

In 1976, the author was sprayed in the face with balanced salt solution by a nurse clearing a syringe. Since the solution produced no conjunctival burning or stinging, the author elected to mix it with local anesthetic solution to see if it would be a less painful diluent for local anesthetics than normal saline and found out that a 1:10 dilution of balanced salt solution and 2% lidocaine caused appreciably no sensation on injection. The 1:10 BSS diluted anesthetic solution was subsequently used to start IVs or as a preliminary injection for skin wheals to precede Van Lint or lid blocks and the infero-temporal injections for eye blocks, and for other regional anesthetic techniques. A painless topical anesthetic was prepared adding one ml of 0.5% proparacaine to 15 ml of BSS.

The Gills/Loyd transconjunctival technique[26] advocated the use of topical proparacaine to anesthetize the conjunctiva and 1% lidocaine solution as a less painful injection to precede injections of bupivacaine. The author substituted his BSS diluted local anesthetic solutions and anesthetized the track to beyond the capsulo-palpebral fascia for the infero-temporal transconjunctival injection, and upon returning the needle to the lid, redirected it in the area of the infraorbital nerve, trying to dissect the preseptal space transconjunctivally through the lid. The transconjunctival route for painlessly anesthetizing the lid for blepharoplasty had been described by Richard Tenzel, and RFH had been using that approach for blepharoplasty anesthesia. The transconjunctival route with lower lid infiltration was a natural addition to the Gills/Loyd technique, and has eliminated the need for a facial nerve block. The painlessness of the Gills/Loyd block encouraged the author to greatly reduce and usually eliminate the use of thiopental for blocks. Since 1985 over 95% of blocks are done with the patient awake and over 98% are pain-free. In 1975, the author substituted a mixture of two parts of 0.75% bupivacaine, one part 2% Mepivacaine® with 1:300,000 epinephrine with 0.5 ml of hyaluronidase solution per ml for the lidocaine/tetracaine mixture that he had previously been using, and has stayed with that mixture ever since; it provides reasonable rapid onset with prolonged analgesia. For blocks in which akinesia is not sought, the author mixes equal parts of the eye block mixture with balanced salt solution. Such a mixture gives very rapid onset of anesthesia and is excellent for procedures like blepharoplasty or intra-orbitally for very anxious patients for photocoagulation; it is painless if preceded by the 1:10 dilution. A sharp 27 gauge 1.25" Monoject needle was used until 1989 (16,000 +/- cases) when the 27 gauge 1.25" BD clear hub needle became available.

Current Technique

The author's current practice is to continually monitor the EKG and BP, make a test injection of 0.2 ml local anesthetic in the skin, start an IV through that skin wheal, place a 24 gauge cannula into a vein, inject 0.3 ml of the dilute local anesthetic intravenously, make a test injection of thiopental (12.5 mg) or midazolam (0.2 mg), and then to make a test injection of local anesthetic alongside the eye with a 1" 30 gauge needle through the everted lower lid (see Figures 1.7 and 1.14) when that is available, or in the same spot on the outside of the lid for tight lids (see Figure 1.8).

Ordinarily no sedation is used except the test injection. Systolic blood pressure in excess of 155 mm Hg is controlled by some combination of sublingual nifedipine, intravenous propranolol or hydralazine, or intravenous sedation.

The 30 gauge 1" needle is introduced at 8:00 (4:00 left eye) down the infero-temporal ATC just inferior to the inferior border of the lateral rectus muscle going through the capsulopalpebral fascia in the adipose tunnel to a depth of 20 mm where 0.5 ml anesthetic in injected. The needle is then withdrawn to the subconjunctiva, redirected towards the infraorbital foramen where 1.25 ml of dilute anesthetic solution is injected preseptally to allow faster diffusion of anesthetic and to make the lid block painless.

After 30 seconds (if a patient needs no allergy check) or up to 10 minutes, a B-D clear hub 27 gauge 1.25" needle is inserted to follow the same pathways, placing the point of the needle at approximately 5-8 mm behind the hind surface of the eye, and 4 ml of local anesthetic solution is injected (3 ml from 1974 to 1978, 3.5 ml until 1990, and 4 ml to date—over 2,000). No brainstem anesthesia, contralateral amaurosis, or unexpected drowsiness have occurred to date. The globe is balloted at the point of 2.5 ml of injection, and is intermittently balloted until the 4 ml has been injected. If there is any increase in intraocular pressure or fullness of the superior lid crease prior to the 4 ml injection, the injection is stopped. The 4 ml is injected at a rate not to exceed 0.5 ml in five seconds. Thus, the injection is done intermittently, 0.5 ml at a time, as learned in principle from Gills and Loyd. The needle is withdrawn back to the conjunctiva and redirected into the preseptal space in the region of the infraorbital foramen where 1.5 ml of the anesthetic is injected at the rate of 0.5 ml/10 seconds, and any injection stopped if the patient feels any sensation. This injection is intended to block the infraorbital nerve, or at least its lid branches, and the zygomatico-facial.

Patients with a small orbit, puffy lids, or elevated intraocular pressure have a bulb placed over the eye after the test dose local anesthetic injection to reduce lid puffiness and intraocular pressure so that the infero-temporal injection will cause less pressure increase.[44] However, for most patients with an average orbit and no history of glaucoma, the main injection follows the test dose injection within two minutes.

After the infero-temporal injection has been completed, the globe is gently massaged for a period of about 1 minute and the orbital compression device (Figure 3.25) placed thereon over a single 2x2; the device applies 20-25 mm pressure to the orbit. The device does not cause a scotoma or visual defect when placed over the globe for one hour in the non-blocked orbit.[75]

At the end of five minutes, range of motion is measured to determine percentage of block of the recti, obliques, levator, and orbicularis. Then the medial pericone injection is done through the medial canthal angle with a 30 gauge 1" needle along the medial ATC in the optical axis parallel to the transverse and sagittal planes with the hub stopped at the frontal plane of the iris (point in the plane of the hind surface). If the superior quadrant structures are primarily unblocked, the medial compartment needle is directed approximately 20° superiorly to facilitate flow into those quadrants. If the inferior compartment seems to be less blocked, then the needle is directed inferiorly about 10°. The compartment is filled until the upper lid crease begins to fill again or until there is a ballottable increase in intraocular pressure, at which point the injection in the medial ATC at the hind surface of the globe is terminated and the needle slowly withdrawn to find the preseptal space where 0.5-2 ml of anesthetic solution is injected (depending upon the state of orbicularis paresis following the five minute check and for those with squinty eyes).

The orbital decompression device is again applied and the eye examined five minutes later. Any significant residual akinesia is then noted and a repeat injection in that quadrant undertaken in another five minutes, if necessary.

The supero-temporal injection is done when necessary (5%) with a 27 or 30 gauge 1" needle in the plane of the lateral limbus walking the roof of the orbit, down past the equator and continuing until it intersects the plane parallel to the hind surface of the eye. The needle is angled approximately 10° towards the optical axis and 10° towards the

Figure 3.25. The bulb end of an irrigation syringe with very thin walls and an indentation in the center is used with a half inch elastic strap to apply pressure of 20 to 25 mmHg against the closed lids over a cotton 2x2. The device allows rapid check of ocular tension and orbital fullness because it can be lifted up, seated on the forehead, and then replaced quickly.

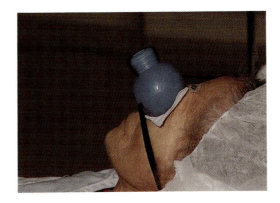

transverse plane to penetrate the septal tissue that connects the levator muscle to the lateral rectus muscle. One expects that the point of the needle will probably be placed medial to the intermuscular septum.

If those three injections do not provide the patient with total akinesia by 20 minutes, then a repeat infero-temporal injection is made with the needle being purposely inserted 3-5 mm more deeply in the orbit.

A 0.3 ml subconjunctival bleb is raised to cover the 10:00 to 2:00 area 5 mm behind the iris.

It is quite variable as to how many supplemental injections need to be made to achieve the desired end point of total akinesia. The medial pericone injection has been a routine for approximately 6,000 cases; prior to that time the injection was made only when needed. In the last 6,000 consecutive cases there have been no cases of hemorrhage or muscle palsy with the 1" 30 gauge needle and the needle placed in the planes of description; a 1" 28 gauge needle would be ideal to allow a bit more feel to the injection.

The author intends to have total akinesia for all patients. Using total akinesia as an end point and purposely making the three quadrant injections for all patients needing enucleation or strabismus surgery the author has been able to assure 99.99% of patients of total absence of sensation during their operative procedure and eight hours of postoperative analgesia.

The author takes care to test vision and the mobility of the globe and notes axial length before any eye block. If the patient has a very large eye or a very small orbit, the infero-temporal needle is placed tangential to the equator of the globe and the injection is made in the infero-temporal compartment, even as far lateral as the insertion of the lateral canthal tendon; if then the needle cannot be placed past the equator as a tangent, the injection is made in the periorbital space. This is necessary in approximately 1% of patients. However, almost always there is plenty of room to move the needle to at least 20° toward the optical axis if not the full 25° that the author intends to use in order to place the needle parallel to the optic nerve (see Figure 1.59).

The author believes that orbital regional anesthesia cannot be learned by looking at written drawings which are often misleading due to perspective and can only be done in a preceptorship role. He encourages visits to his facility to observe the described technique.

JASWANT SINGH PANNU, MD
Pannu Eye Institute, Fort Lauderdale, Florida

Single Injection Peribulbar Technique for Instant Sight[SM] Cataract Surgery

Quick rehabilitation following surgery is the aim of all surgeons.

For the last three years I have been practicing *instant sight*[SM] cataract surgery. With this procedure the patient sees immediately upon completion of surgery and goes without a patch. This is of special significance in a patient with one eye. The following steps are taken to accomplish *instant sight.*

1. *Short Acting Anesthetic*

   1 or 2% Xylocaine with adrenaline and Wydase is used. The anesthetic wears off by the end of the procedure and patients are able to open and close their eyes.

2. *Peribulbar Injection* (illustrated in Figures 3.26 to 3.31)

   My peribulbar technique gives satisfactory anesthetic yet does not block conduction through the optic nerve making it possible for the patient to see upon completion of the procedure.

3. *No Sub-Conjunctival Injection*

   No sub conjunctival antibiotics or steroid injections are given. Although this is not an essential step for *instant sight,* sub-conjunctival injection balloons the conjunctiva making it uncomfortable for the patient to blink.

In the last 10 years I have used single injection peribulbar technique in 3,000 cases with excellent results. During this time the following modifications have been made to make it a safer procedure.

1. *No Long Needles*

   In the first 200 cases I used 1″ or longer needle with great success. This was followed by respiratory arrests in 2 patients immediately following injection. Both patients recovered. One was lost to followup and the other had cataract extraction done using peribulbar technique with a shorter needle (5/8″). It seems the long needle may have penetrated the optic nerve sheath at the apex injecting the anesthetic in the CNS. Since switching to a short needle no such complications have occurred.

2. *No Injection in Upper Lid Area*

   Originally injections were made in the upper lid area using the supra orbital notch as a guide. The needle was advanced lateral to the supra orbital notch along the roof of the orbit and the anesthetic injected in the upper lid area. Sometimes the resulting upper lid ptosis lasted for days or weeks. This was unacceptable and so the site of injection was switched to lower lid area.

3. *Anesthetic Mixture*

   Initially a mixture of Marcaine and Xylocaine was used giving a long lasting anesthesia. With *instant sight* a short acting anesthetic is used. At first it was thought that without Marcaine the patients may complain of pain. This has not happened. During corneal transplant and other prolonged procedures Marcaine is used.

4. *Amount of Anesthetic*

   Originally 8 to 10 ml of anesthetic mixture was used to completely paralyze the eye. Now 4 to 5 ml of Xylocaine with adrenaline and Wydase is used and this gives

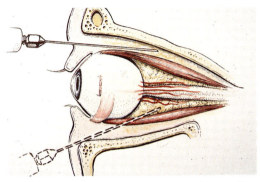

Figure 3.26. Anatomical location for needles for peribulbar and retrobulbar anesthesia. Please compare with figure 3.27.

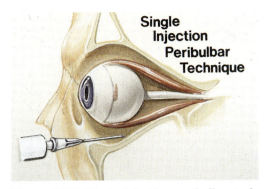

Figure 3.27. Single injection peribulbar technique.

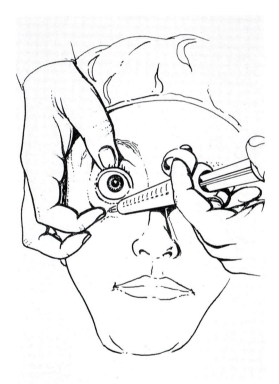

Figure 3.28. Injection site for the Pannu block. Note that the eye is kept wide open.

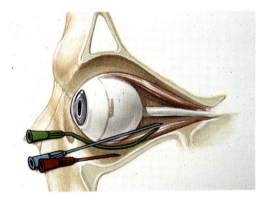

Figure 3.29. Comparison on a model of a retrobulbar and a Straus curved needle.

satisfactory anesthesia. Patient comfort during surgery and not the muscle paralysis is used as the end point. Eye movement during surgery is tolerated except when doing corneal transplant when 8 to 9 ml of anesthetic is used.

5. *No Massage or Wait*

Following injection there is no massaging of the eye or waiting period before start of operation.

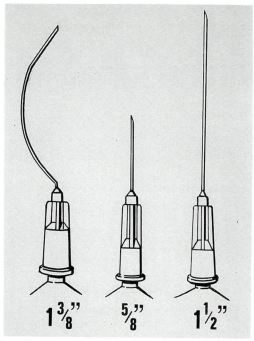

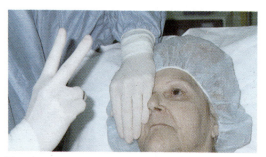

Figure 3.31. Following the injection of 4 ml of 2% Xylocaine with adrenaline and Wydase. The patient's vision is checked and the patient is still able to recognize fingers. Thus the block does not produce absence of vision. Akinesia is not expected.

Figure 3.30. The relative size of a curved and a 1 1/2″ needle.

Complications

1. *Respiratory Arrest*
   In 3,000 cases two respiratory arrests were seen following injection using a 1″ needle. No such complication has occurred with a shorter needle (5/8″).
2. *Ptosis*
   A few cases of ptosis which lasted for several days were seen with injections in the upper lid area. Since switching to the lower lid site of injection this has not been a problem.
3. *Sub-Conjunctival Hemorrhage*
   The only complication in the last 2,000 cases has been occasional small sub conjunctival hemorrhage from the injection.

Present Technique

Four to 5 ml of Xylocaine (1 or 2%) mixed with adrenaline and Wydase is injected with a 5/8″ 25 or 27 gauge needle. The site of injection is the temporal lower lid area using the inferior orbital rim as a guideline.

The needle is advanced touching the floor of the orbit and pointing away from the globe. 4-5 ml of anesthetic is injected. No massaging or waiting period is necessary. This gives satisfactory anesthesia during surgery and wears off soon after the completion of the procedure (Figure 3.32).

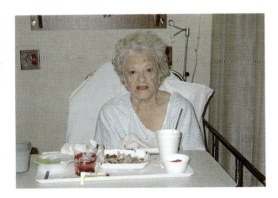

Figure 3.32. Patient alert at the completion of surgery without an eye patch.

JEFFREY G. STRAUS, MD
Straus/Azar Medical Surgical Laser Eye Center
Metairle and Gretna, Louisiana

Retrobulbar Block:
Technique and Needle

The Straus needle and technique were developed to improve the safety of retrobulbar injection. Certainly everyone would agree that retrobulbar anesthesia is a very effective technique. However, concerns about improved safety have escalated in the last few years secondary to an increased number of complications. While peribulbar injection is not a new technique, application of the peribulbar injection for the provision of regional anesthesia for eye surgery has certainly gained increased popularity in the last several years. Again, this is because doctors have sought to reduce the risks associated with retrobulbar anesthesia. However, there are several advantages of retrobulbar anesthesia versus peribulbar anesthesia. First, there is a higher rate of adequate block with retrobulbar anesthesia, primarily because the elaborate musculo-fibrous septa outside the muscle cone, as elucidated by Dr. Koornneef, create a barrier to the spread of peribulbar anesthetic.

Secondly, an increased rate of adequate block results in an increased rate of single intraorbital injection with a resultant decreased risk of hemorrhage and decreased risk of perforation of the globe. And, if an adequate block is obtained with peribulbar injection, the onset of anesthesia and akinesia is prolonged. Retrobulbar anesthetized patients are unlikely to complain about microscope lights. Any decrease of intraoperative stimuli is advantageous.

Lastly, the larger volume of anesthetic generally used with the peribulbar technique may be a problem. Immediately following peribulbar injection the orbit often becomes very tense and the eye is often very hard. Although transient, this pressure rise is worrisome for patients with small blood vessel disease and/or compromised optic nerve function, a large number of geriatric patients, and those most likely to be undergoing eye surgery. The number of resultant postoperative visual field defects from these transient intraocular pressure spikes is unknown.

It seemed that the simplest way to reduce the risk of ocular perforation was to a curved needle. Certainly a curved needle could negotiate a globe with less risk of perforation than a straight needle. Clearly, ocular perforation is one of the worst possible complications of retrobulbar anesthesia. However, simply using a curved needle to get to the retrobulbar space does nothing to protect the optic nerve from direct trauma or possible subarachnoid injection. Therefore, the design of the needle and technique were modified for retrobulbar injection.

The proximal portion of the needle is curved (Figures 3.33, 3.34). The straight distal portion of the needle is10 mm long and approaches the longitudinal axis of the hub at an angle of 30°. The bevel is toward the sclera. The overall length of the needle is 34 mm or approximately 1 3/8 inches. It is produced in 25 gauge and 23 gauge versions.

The two-step placement method is as follows (Figure 3.35 through 3.37): (1) The straight distal portion of the needle is passed posteriorly close to the globe in the inferotemporal quadrant of the orbit. Once the straight portion is passed to the beginning of the curve at the surface of the conjunctiva, the anesthetist is assured that the tip of the

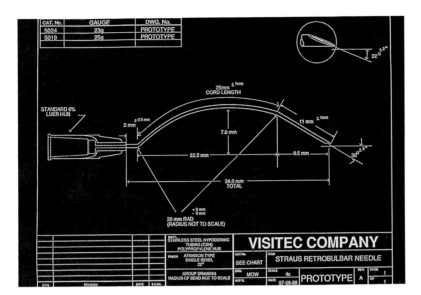

Figure 3.33. Diagram of the Straus needle.

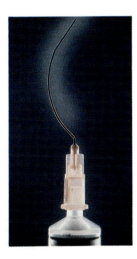

Figure 3.34. Photograph of the Straus needle.

needle is posterior to the equator of the globe. (2) The curve of the needle is followed by the syringe until the tip of the needle is within the muscle cone. Since the needle does not contact the globe and the orbital contents are flaccid, there is very little resistance to passage and penetration of the anterior portion of the muscle cone (which is the thickest portion, according to Dr. Koornneef).

The needle is withdrawn reversing the two steps of placement. The injecting hand moves nasally while removing the curved portion and away from the patient anteriorly while removing the straight portion.

In Figures 3.38, 3.39, it can be clearly seen that the straight distal portion of the needle is inferior to the optic foramen and the 30° angle of that portion of the needle approximately parallels the intra-orbital segment of the optic nerve. Thus subarachnoid injection or trauma to the optic nerve is highly unlikely.

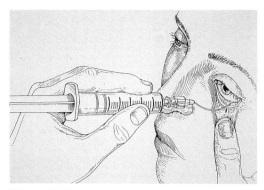

Figure 3.35.

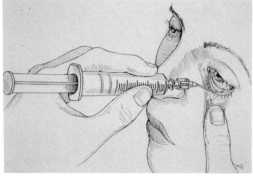

Figure 3.36.

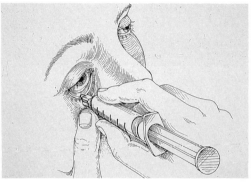

Figure 3.37.

Figures 3.35 through 3.37. Demonstration of the two-step placement method.

In Figures 3.40, 3.41 the two-step resistance placement method is demonstrated on a patient. Comparison of the differences in approach to the retrobulbar space shows that when a straight needle is used, a triangular plane of intraocular space is violated, while with the Straus needle, only a curvilinear space is violated (Figures 3.42, 3.43). There is less stress on the tissue that is violated since the globe is not displaced either by the shaft of the needle or by the anesthetist's finger pressing on the lower lid as is often done to facilitate passage of a straight needle. Since the globe is not displaced, the intraorbital vessels remain flaccid and are thus less likely to rupture if contacted by the needle.

While advancing the tip of the straight needle to the retrobulbar space, it is clear how ocular perforation can occur, furthermore, it is apparent that the tip of the needle is approaching the optic nerve at approximately a 45° angle. The Straus needle does not pass inferiorly to the globe rather it passes around the globe inferotemporally and the straight distal portion enters the muscle cone inferior and parallel to the optic nerve.

In Figure 3.44, the needle can be seen coursing around the globe. The straight distal portion is within the cone just medial to the lateral rectus muscle. it is inferotemporal and parallel to the optic nerve.

To date, more than 10,000 blocks have been performed with the Straus needle and technique. There have been no reports of penetration or perforation of the globe, subarachnoid injection, or optic nerve trauma, although there has been one report of retrobulbar hemorrhage (*Ophthalmology Times*, Jan. 15, 1992). Indeed, with proper technique, the risk of perforation of the globe is extremely low for most eyes since the arc of curvature of the needle is greater than that of any eye 30 mm or less in axial length and

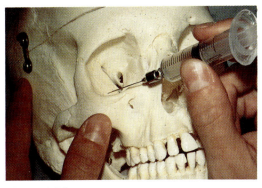
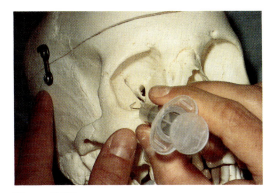

Figure 3.38.   **Figure 3.39.**

Figures 3.38 and 3.39. Demonstration of the two-step placement method on a human skull.

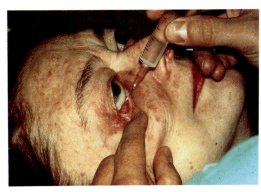
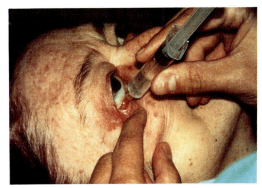

Figure 3.40.   **Figure 3.41.**

Figures 3.40 and 3.41. Demonstration of the two-step resistance placement method on a patient.

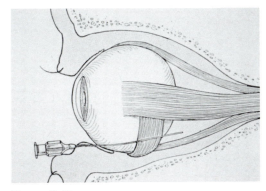
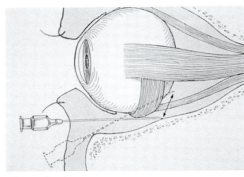

Figure 3.42.   **Figure 3.43.**

Figures 3.42 and 3.43. The difference in approach to the retrobulbar space when using a straight needle and when using a Straus needle.

because the tip of the needle is posterior to the equator of the globe before it is directed medially.

Editors' Comment

The Straus needle with its curved and straight segment is a unique mechanical solution to a long held concept of curved needles for anesthesia in the orbit. Since the globe is curved, why not make a curved needle to follow the globe back to the retrobulbar space. Through the years, a number of people have used curved needle technique (Braun cites three before 1910: Haab, Mende, and Seidel). The technique was re-invented by Jan Worst of Holland, Fred Hill of Hattiesburg, Mississippi and Dr. Buttery in Australia.[62]

The rapid onset of akinesia when a curved needle is placed 5 mm behind the eye is one of those clinching points of argument that there is, in fact, a "central or oculomotor" compartment containing the ciliary nerve and surrounding the optic nerve; this central space helps maintain higher concentration of anesthetic as it moves back to the orbital apex to block branches of the oculomotor nerve. It is surprising that more persons doing sub-Tenon's injections have not inadvertently found this space. Have they failed to note the extent of paresis from sub-Tenon's injections?

Hustead has watched Dr. Fred Hill do 14 consecutive blocks with absolute akinesia at the end of three minutes using 4 ml of a mixture of 2% lidocaine and 0.5% bupivacaine—and the needle was not more than 5 mm behind the eye. Dr. Hill has given up the curved needle technique following two cases of brainstem apnea, although neither patient suffered damage to the optic nerve. Such a potential is high. Note in Figure 1.31 what a large area of subarachnoid space exists along the optic nerve about 5 mm behind the hind surface of the eye. This space can be much larger in some persons. A short beveled needle could discharge the entire content in the CSF.

Dr. Straus believes the straight segment after the curve will prevent this complication and so far it has not been reported in 10,000 uses of the needle. Dr. Hill had done 8,000 before he had two cases within three weeks, but his needle was not identical, only very similar to Dr. Straus' needle.

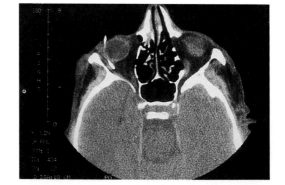

Figure 3.44. An in vivo CT evaluation of the Straus needle which was performed at Tulane Medical Center in New Orleans.

SPENCER P. THORNTON, MD
Baptist Hospital, Nashville, Tennessee

Ocular Anesthesia with the
Thornton Retrobulbar Needle

Difficulties with retrobulbar anesthesia with standard and blunted retrobulbar needles have included peribulbar and retrobulbar hemorrhage, lacerations and penetration of the globe and damage to the optic nerve.[63-71] These and other complications have occurred with both disposable and nondisposable retrobulbar needles because of the cutting edges of these needles. Blunting of the tips does not reduce the danger of these complications and in fact makes penetration of the skin more difficult and painful.

The Thornton Needle (available from Alcon Surgical) was developed to avoid these complications and facilitate the induction of ocular anesthesia with minimal discomfort and maximum effect. Up until the present time, general anesthesia, with all of its risks, was the only reliable alternative to retrobulbar injection with standard or blunted retrobulbar needles.[28,72]

Description of the Needle

The Thornton Needle (Figures 3.45a,b) was designed to eliminate cutting edges, tapering to an ultra-sharp smooth tip which enters the skin with minimal resistance.[12] The edges are rounded and the 15 degree bevel tip is designed to run truer through tissue when properly placed beneath the orbital rim. The needle is 25 gauge, thin-walled (0.08 mm) with all edges rounded and highly polished to decrease tissue resistance and injection pressure. An indexing "guide" tab on the hub of the needle indicates to the surgeon the back or pointed side of the needle which is the side away from the hole in the beveled surface of the tip. It should be remembered that the beveled "hole" side should be toward the eye on any peribulbar or retrobulbar injection.

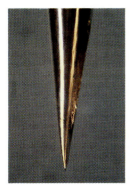

Figure 3.45a. Side view of the Thornton needle.

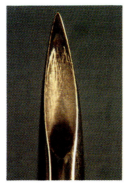

Figure 3.45b. Front or bevel view of the Thornton needle.

Technique

The "posterior peribulbar" approach is recommended instead of the standard retrobulbar technique which attempts to place the tip of the injection needle within the muscle cone behind the globe. Since with posterior peribulbar anesthesia the injection needle does not penetrate the muscle cone, there is little chance of injuring the optic nerve or retrobulbar blood vessels.

Posterior peribulbar anesthesia can be administered either above or below the eye entering adjacent to the orbital rim. In the superior approach the needle is introduced just below the orbital rim lateral to the temporal edge of the superior rectus muscle (Figure 3.46) and the needle tip is directed 45 degrees upward (Figure 3.47) toward the orbital roof away from the globe and the muscle cone until the needle is introduced approximately 1 cm or until the roof of the orbit is gently touched (Figure 3.48 & 3.49). The back of the needle should be aimed away from the globe.

The needle is then redirected toward the back of the head (Figure 3.50) and slowly advanced until the posterior wall of the orbit is encountered behind the globe (Figure 3.51). There is no attempt to enter the muscle cone. The tab on the hub of the needle is

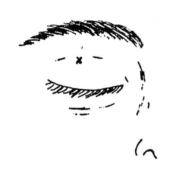

Figure 3.46. Needle introduced just below orbital rim lateral to temporal edge of the superior rectus muscle.

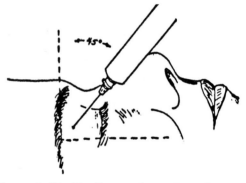

Figure 3.47. Needle tip directed 45 degrees upward toward orbital roof.

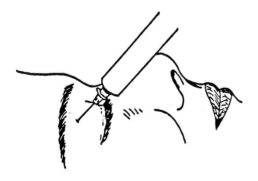

Figure 3.48.

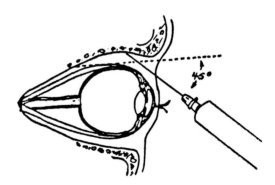

Figure 3.49.

Figures 3.48 and 3.49. Needle introduced approximately 1cm or until roof of orbit is gently touched.

directed away from the globe so that the point is away from the globe (that is so that the hole of the needle is toward the globe). In other words, the needle should be inserted aiming up toward the roof of the orbit for about 1 cm to get past the equator of the globe then aimed straight back (Figure 3.49-3.52). The anesthetic mixture is injected at this point (Figure 3.53).

A 5 to 6 ml solution of 0.75% Marcaine and 4% Xylocaine with Wydase can achieve satisfactory anesthesia. With this injection one should see some ballooning of the upper lid with resulting lid block and even some retrograde 5th and 7th nerve block avoiding the necessity of additional injections. An orbital pressure device should be applied over the eye for at least 20 minutes to allow spread of the anesthetic throughout the orbit and orbicularis.

If the infraorbital approach is preferred, the needle is inserted through the skin just above the inferior orbital rim just lateral to the temporal margin of the inferior rectus and directed slightly downward toward the orbital floor away from the globe for about 1 cm, the needle is redirected directly toward the back of the orbit. Anesthesia may be injected as the needle is advanced. With this technique there is little danger of penetrating the globe or the muscle cone.

Since the needle is directed away from the eye during insertion, there is less chance of perforating it. This injection method avoids the anterior and posterior ciliary

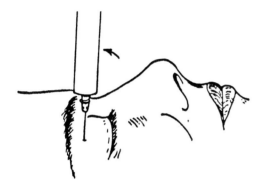

Figure 3.50. Needle redirected to the back of the head.

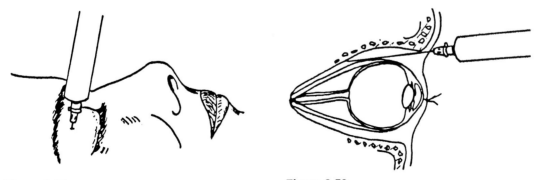

Figure 3.51.   **Figure 3.52**
Figures 3.51 and 3.52. Needle advanced until the posterior wall of the orbit is encountered.

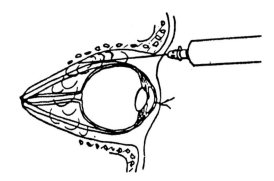

Figure 3.53. The anesthetic mixture is injected at this point.

vessels as well as the vortex veins. With the hub's tab as a guide and the hypotraumatic tip passing outside the muscle cone there is less chance of penetrating the optic nerve, and with no cutting edges, the chance of retrobulbar hemorrhage is minimal.

Only one injection is needed through either the upper or lower lid and no additional lid block (Van Lint, O'Brien or Nadbath) is necessary.

Editors' Comment

Dr. Thornton refers to his technique as "posterior peribulbar" anesthesia, although the needle point is placed in the mid-orbit. The technique of walking along the orbital roof in order to get past the equator of the eye is beautifully demonstrated. The needle, in Figure 3.52 is placed 10° inferior to the transverse plane. The hub of the needle is placed at 1 mm anterior to the frontal plane of the corneal surface, and the point of the needle is placed 1 mm posterior to the hind surface of the eye. Therefore, the needle length would have been 27 mm.

Figure 1.59e is a computer reconstruction of the placement of this needle in which the point of the needle is placed 1 mm posterior to the hind surface of the eye, and the hub of a 25 mm needle intersects the frontal plane of the limbus in the parasagittal plane of the limbus. If the needle point lies external to the two layers of intermuscular septum, then a periorbital injection would ensue. If the needle traverses the intermuscular septum, then an intraconal injection would occur.

Various authors have used this superior-temporal approach to obtain ocular anesthesia. Dr. Kelman uses a bent needle to obtain reliable insertion into the muscle cone from the superior-temporal position. Hustead and Hamilton use the supero-temporal quadrant as a supplementary injection for those people in whom infero-temporal or medial placement does not provide akinesia of the superior rectus or levator muscle.

Hustead stands behind the patient, as does Dr. Thornton, which takes the needle and all action out of the patient's view. Both Hustead and Hamilton have the patient's eye open as soon as the needle is placed through the upper lid in contact with the roof. The needle is then moved beyond the equator of the eye with the lids open to ensure no unexpected contact with the globe occurs.

Injection in the supero-temporal quadrant is an effective way to block the frontal nerve and the lacrimal nerve and their conjunctival branches. Injection of 5 to 6 ml in this quadrant has quite variable effects at producing occular akinesia and obtaining good block of the ciliary ganglion and nerves.

The intermuscular septum is very tenuous proceeding posterior from 5 mm anterior to the hind surface of the eye, making an avenue of easy ingress into the mid-orbit anterior to the cone—and for ingress of solution.

Therefore, unless a needle is angled 20° to the optical axis or the shaft bent, or a longer needle is used to cause the point to enter the muscle cone, the injection will often produce very little akinesia.

In a visit to Dr. Thornton in 1989, the variability of akinesia was noted. However, this in no way interfered with Dr. Thornton's exquisite surgery or patient satisfaction.

The Thornton needle, with its 15° bevel and polished edges, is an engineer's dream in making a beveled needle into a non-cutting but non-coring instrument. However, when Hustead used a series of needles, he was unable to introduce a third of the needles without causing rotation of the globe because the tissue would adhere to the shaft of the needle and prevent the needle sliding in its tunnel path when the needle was inserted about 10 mm in periorbital tissue containing no significant septa.

The puncture made by the needle may be so small that tissue just cannot slide back except on the most highly polished surface. This factor could be minimized by slight changes in the point of the needle, more polish to the shaft of the needle, or siliconizing the shaft of the needle, as is done with most disposable needles. Hustead was able to pass a 27 gauge needle down the hole made by the 25 gauge Thornton needle without the septa adhering to the shaft of the 27 gauge needle.

HAI-SHIUH WANG, MD
Eye Care Associates, Youngstown, Ohio

Peribulbar Anesthesia

Local Anesthesia Agents

Ten cc of 0.75% bupivacaine (Marcaine) are mixed with 1 cc hyaluronidase (Wydase) in a 10 cc plastic syringe. The needle is 1 1/2 inches long with a sharp tip (Figure 3.54).

Injection Technique

The orbital frame is divided into three compartments by two vertical lines (Figure 3.55).

At the point of the lateral vertical line, the skin of the lower lid between the globe and orbital rim, a small wheal is raised with an anesthetic solution (Figure 3.56). Since the skin is quite sensitive, an anesthetic here allows the remainder of the procedure to proceed with relatively little discomfort.

While the eye stares straight forward, the needle penetrates perpendicular to the skin and into the orbit about one inch (Figures 3.57a,b,c) between the lateral and inferior rectus muscles. The plunger of the syringe is slightly withdrawn to ensure it is not in a vessel.

The index and middle finger of the fellow hand presses the inferior sulcus of the lower lid while 6 cc anesthetic solution is injected without moving the needle (Figures 3.58a, b).

With the pressure of the index and middle fingers, the injected anesthetic solution at the inferior lateral compartment of the posterior orbit will flow toward the nasal and superior compartments of the posterior orbit, and later diffuse forward to paralyze the orbicularis muscles and all sensory nerve fibers (Figure 3.59).

Often, toward the end of injection, drooping of the upper lid, bulging of the superior orbital sulcus, and mydriasis are noted (Figure 3.60).

After the needle is withdrawn, the lid is taped closed. A Honan Balloon® is applied at the recommended 35 mmHg for 10 minutes on and five minutes off. This is done twice (Figure 3.61).

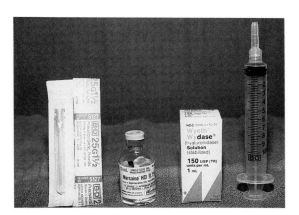

Figure 3.54. Anesthetic solution, syringe and needle.

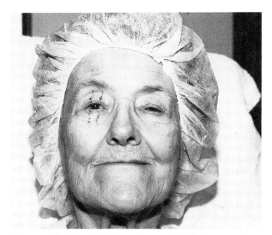

Figure 3.55. Divide the orbital frame into three compartments with two vertical lines.

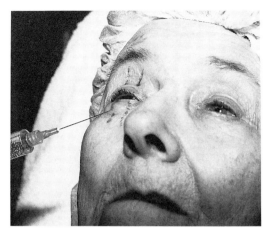

Figure 3.56. A small wheal is raised in the skin with an anesthetic agent at the injection site of the lateral line of the lower lid between the globe and orbital rim.

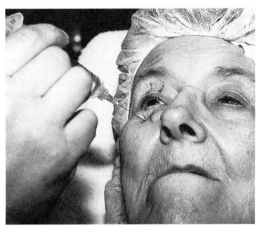

Figure 3.57a.

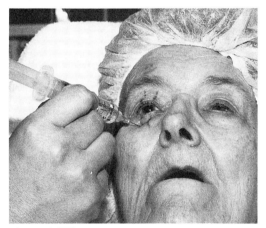

Figure 3.57b.

Figures 3.57a, b. While the patient stares forward, the needle penetrates perpendicular to the skin and into the orbit about one inch.

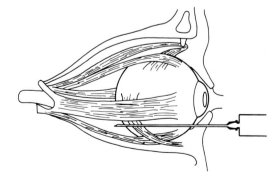

Figure 3.57c. Schematic lateral views of the needle position between the lateral and inferior rectus muscle, the tip of the needle is placed at the posterior border of the globe.

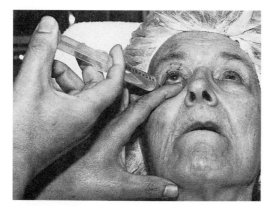

Figure 3.58a.   **Figure 3.58b.**

Figure 3.58a, b. Illustration of hands and fingers position. While pressing the inferior sulcus of the lower lid with the left index and middle fingers, inject 6 cc of anesthetic solution with the right hand.

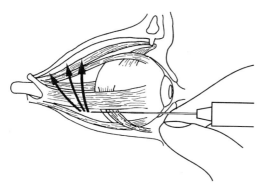

Figure 3.59. Schematic drawing of the injected anesthetic solution diffused from the inferior temporal compartment toward the superior, nasal, and inferior compartments of the posterior orbit while the inferior sulcus of the lower lid is held and pressed by fingers.

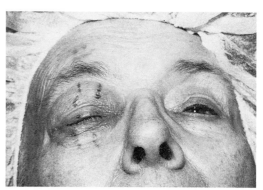

Figure 3.60. Noted progressive drooping of the upper lid or bulging of the superior sulcus of the upper lid at the end of the injection.

The anesthesia and akinesia of the lids and globe should be rechecked prior to surgery by following movement of the globe and orbicularis muscle action (Figure 3.62).

If inadequate anesthesia or akinesia results, most often in the superior and medial rectus muscle, a supplementary injection is given. In my experience, 20 to 30% of cases require a supplementary injection.

When the superior and/or medial rectus muscles are incompletely blocked, the injection site of the supranasal quadrant of the orbit should be between the globe and the orbit rim. When only the superior rectus muscle is incompletely blocked, the injection site should be as close to the nasal border of the muscle as possible (Figure 3.63a,b); and when only the medial rectus muscle is incompletely blocked, the injection site should be as close to the superior border of the muscle as possible (Figure 3.63c,d). Avoid direct injection of the muscle itself because it could cause hemorrhaging or muscle damage. The needle should be inserted one inch deep (Figure 3.64), usually injecting 1 cc of an anesthetic solution is adequate.

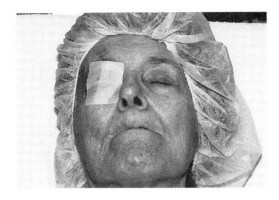

Figure 3.61a. The lid is taped closed to avoid damage of the anesthetic cornea from an orbital pressure device.

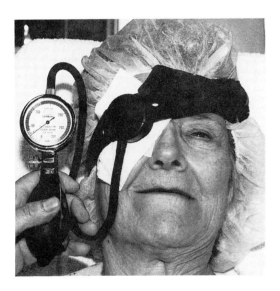

Figure 3.61b. A Honan balloon® is applied at the recommended pressure of 35 mmHg for 10 minutes.

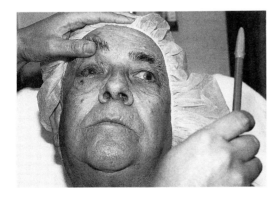

Figure 3.62. Prior to surgery, akinesia of the external ocular muscles and the orbicularis muscles should be tested by following the movement of the eye and squeezing the lids.

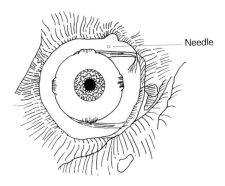

Figure 3.63a.

Figures 3.63a, b.   The needle position for incomplete akinesia of the superior rectus muscle is near the nasal border of the superior rectus muscle, not directly at the muscle.

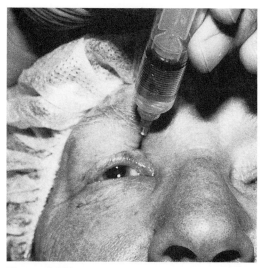

Figure 3.63b.

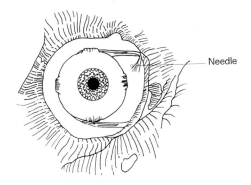

Figure 3.63c.

Figures 3.63c, d.   The needle position for incomplete akinesia of the medial rectus muscle is near the superior border of the medial rectus muscle.

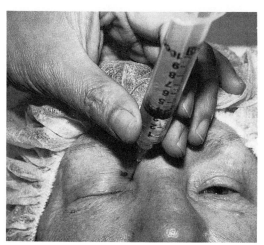

Figure 3.63d.

Editors' Comment

Dr. Wang in 1988, published his version of "peribulbar technique." Four line drawings established where needles should enter the orbit and where their points should lie. An injection in the supero-nasal quadrant of 4 ml of 0.75% bupivacaine was followed in two to three minutes by an injection of 4 ml in the infero-temporal compartment.[32] The location of the point of the 1 1/2" 25 gauge needle was clearly marked on the diagrams, and that point was at 1 mm behind the hind surface of the eye.

The injection site of the infero-temporal injection was made confusing by the line-drawing which showed a lateral view of the globe with the superior oblique muscle and trochlea still in evidence; however, if one ignored the problem of artistic presentation, one could ascertain where the infero-temporal injection was to go.

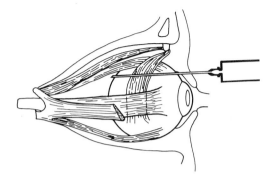

Figure 3.64. The schematic superior view of the needle position of the superior nasal injection is between the superior and medial rectus muscle and should be inserted one inch deep.

The block was checked at about 15 minutes after the two injections and was supplemented by a repeat peribulbar injection of 2 ml or by an injection directly to the acting muscle.

Dr. Wang has now significantly changed the block and has improved his graphics. A 6 ml injection is now done in the infero-temporal quadrant, and the supero-nasal quadrant is only used as a supplementary injection. Approximate spread of anesthetic from the injection sites was not undertaken on the computerized drawings of Figure 1.59 because of space restraints. However, the reader can make a close approximation by comparing his injection sites with those analyzed in Figures 1.59b-i.

An analysis of his photographs of actual blocks may not give a true perspective because of camera angle and the angle of the patient's face, nor can we deduce where the point of the needle actually goes because in the individual patient the axial length of the eye was not noted. However, the best guess puts the needle shaft approximately 20° toward the optical axis instead of being parallel to the sagittal plane in the infero-nasal injection, assuming an axial length of 24 mm.

In the supero-nasal injection, the point was angled approximately 10° toward the optical axis. In both cases, needle point is close to the plane of the hind surface of the eye because of the amount of needle shaft which has not entered the skin. Angulation of 20° infero-temporal and 10° supero-nasal still allows the needle to move within the space between the muscles and central to them. The needle point should be a safe distance away from any vital structures. Angling toward the optical axis from any peribulbar skin site would increase the risk of perforation

Dr. Wang encourages the use of a 1 1/2″ needle to keep much of needle outside the plane of the cornea so that the amount of needle passing alongside the eye can be judged. The patient was asked to stare straight ahead to give the anesthetist perspective thereby obtaining some indication if the needle were in capsulo-palpebral fascia close to the sclera.

If the needles were inserted 5 to 8 mm more than they are diagrammed, the block could produce entirely different clinical responses; but, even an additional 5 mm of needle insertion should not place the needle points in dangerous areas of the mid-orbit.

TOPICAL ANESTHESIA

Richard A. Fichman, MD
Fichman Eye Center, Manchester, Connecticut

Fichman Technique for Topical Anesthesia

In 1991 it became apparent that topical anesthesia could be a boon in intraocular surgery, partly because the building blocks for its use were already present. Discussions with other ophthalmologists and clinicians and personal experience indicated that some basic, necessary elements were already established.

Those elements included the proven knowledge that patients could be trusted to fixate on a target during surgery; that phacoemulsification could be performed even when patients' eyes were capable of movement; that the cornea and conjunctiva could be anesthetized properly with topical anesthesia; and that the iris could be manipulated under topical anesthesia (already seen in YAG and argon iridotomies and in holmium procedures).

During the summer of 1991, I began lowering the dose of lidocaine given in my blocks from 4 cc to 1 cc. Ocular movement was possible, but generally patients responded well to instructions regarding fixation. Even when eye movement occurred, it was generally mild and the phaco tip's leverage inside the eye made it very difficult for gross eye movements.

In October 1991, I performed my first case of cataract surgery under topical anesthesia. The case went well, and from that time on topical has been my anesthesia of choice for most cataract surgeries.

Assessment

Perhaps more than in any other technique a careful assessment of the patient is imperative in the use of topical anesthesia for intraocular surgery. This can begin with a conversation in the holding area ranging from mundane topics such as how the patient slept to asking the patient whether they are anxious or how they are feeling in general. This is a very basic technique and can provide the first clues as to whether the patient is a good candidate for topical anesthesia and whether supplemental IV sedation will be necessary.

A patient whose voice is tremulous, who avoids the surgeon's glance, or admits to being nervous should probably have a small dose of IV sedation, preferably before entering the operating room.

On the contrary, a patient who seems confident and calm may be one who will not require any supplemental anesthesia.

Experience suggests that these factors can change at any time during the perioperative period, however this minute or two spent with the patient pre-operatively is often adjunct in administration of topical anesthesia.

Pre-Operative Regimen

Once in the operating room, a concerted effort is made to make the patient as comfortable as possible: warm blankets, pillows under the knees, or neck can be very helpful in preventing future problems. It is difficult to discern midway through the procedure why the patient is restless and it is not unusual to find that discomfort due to positioning, being cold, or having to void. These problems make the patient less compliant, and movement associated with these problems can lead the physician to assume that the patient is having ocular discomfort.

After the patient is comfortable a conversation is maintained during the pre-operative period. It is useful to note during this time the patient's reactions to several minor tests. When the blood pressure cuff squeezes the arm some patients barely note the event, other patients are extremely vocal about their discomfort. Similarly, the placement of EKG leads and nasal cannulae can give some insight as to the patient's pain threshold and profile. This is useful for two reasons: it serves as a preview of how the patient will relate to other events during surgery and this may be the first clue that supplemental anesthesia may be useful.

At this point, 1 drop of .5% tetracaine is instilled into the operative eye patient being warned in advance that this will sting and is asked to close their eye and count to ten slowly. After this the patient is usually comfortable and the eye is prepared according to the surgeon's preference. After the drape is placed, the lid speculum is placed in the eye. This is another point at which the patient's anxiety level and also the effects of the topical anesthesia can be judged. If the patient is fighting the speculum, the ophthalmologist should determine if this is due to anxiety or pain. If it is due to anxiety, gentle reassurance should be offered and the patient's anxiety level monitored for the next two minutes to determine if supplemental anesthesia will be necessary.

With the speculum in place, two additional drops of .5% tetracaine are administered. If the patient notes that it stings, then it is wise to wait approximately one minute and re-instill additional drops until the stinging has subsided.

The microscope is set on its lowest illumination and the patient is told in advance that they will be seeing a very bright light. The vast majority of patients will be comfortable with this. A minute or so is sometimes required for the patient to be comfortable with the intensity of the light, however, in a very small minority of patients (less than 1%) this situation is unacceptable and they will move their eyes and head to avoid the light.

If this situation occurs, it is wise to abandon topical anesthesia and to prepare a retrobulbar block. This will not only provide akinesia but also eliminate photophobia. This block can be administered with the drapes in place through the inferior cul-de-sac. For the 99% of patients in whom this does not occur, the procedure can begin.

A .3 forceps is used to test conjunctival anesthesia; first by merely pressing against conjunctiva and sclera, later by grasping the conjunctiva if a peritomy is to be performed during the surgery. Many patients say they feel some degree of pressure once forceps touch the globe. However, upon further questioning they indicate this is not painful, and if they are advised that this is normal, they will readily adapt to the situation.

At this point it is important to advise the patient that should this feeling of pressure ever become uncomfortable during the procedure or if pain should develop it is perfectly reasonable to notify the surgeon and that medicines will be administered to immediately alleviate the discomfort.

A dialogue querying the patient's status concerning anxiety should be done every three to five minutes during the procedure.

Surgical Technique

Once the surgeon is comfortable with the patient's anxiety level and anesthesia, the patient is asked to look down. This is one of the bonuses of topical anesthetic as it affords excellent exposure for either a corneal incision or scleral tunnel. If a peritomy and scleral incision are performed, in a small percentage of cases, the patient will become uncomfortable with excessive manipulation of conjunctiva and/or sclera or during cautery. A micropore sponge soaked with .5% tetracaine can be placed over the area of the incision for 30 seconds to one minute, and will alleviate any pain from this part of the procedure. Entry into the cornea can be made following this process (Figure 3.65).

Neither bridle sutures nor a second instrument is used to fixate the eye. The patient is instructed to look down during the creation of the incision and capsulorhexis. The incision is begun just anterior to the limbal conjunctival junction. The corneal incision is made in three stages to avoid the creation of a loose flap of conjunctiva (Figure 3.66a,b). An incision is made with a keratome in the center of the proposed incision site, dissecting down. The keratome is withdrawn and moved to one edge of the initial wound and another stab is made in the same plane to widen the incision. The keratome is withdrawn and the other side of the incision is widened. The anterior chamber entry is made by placing the keratome back at the position of the initial stab, tilting the point down and advancing the blade (Figure 3.67a,b,c and Figure 3.68a,b).

Once the anterior chamber has been entered viscoelastic is injected into the anterior chamber. The patient is asked to slowly look up towards the microscope light. If a cystotome is in the anterior chamber it is useful to remove it before asking the patient to look up. The cystotome can be reintroduced once the patient is fixating on the microscope light. During capsulorhexis it is important to instruct the patient to fixate directly on the light and a dialogue at this point is very helpful.

Reassurance is offered throughout the capsulorhexis. For the novice, it is useful to use .2 forceps to help stabilize the eye during capsulorhexis. After capsulorhexis is completed, hydrodissection and hydrodelineation are carried out. During these procedures stretching of the zonules may occur abruptly and the patient may indicate a twinge of pain or the surgeon may note that the patient squeezes on the lid speculum. This is an important observation. Although it is short-lived several episodes like this can tend to make the patient non-compliant, therefore, in this type of patient when the phacoemulsification tip is inserted into the eye the bottle may be lowered such that in position one an immediate burst of fluid will not result in stretching the zonules.

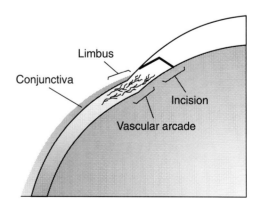

Figure 3.65. The two-plane valve construction of the corneal wound is begun anterior to the limbal conjunctival reflection.

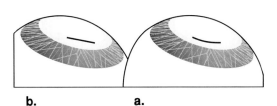

Figure 3.66a, b. Making the corneal incision as a single stab wound can result in an arcuate incision (a) that leaves a flap of tissue postoperatively. The three-stage incision results in a self-sealing linear wound that closes cleanly (b).

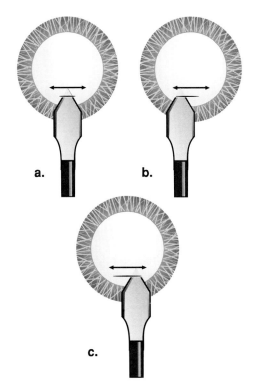

Figure 3.67a, b, c. An initial stab is made in the center of the incision site (a), dissecting about one-third corneal depth. The keratome is withdrawn and moved to one edge of the initial wound (b) and another stab is made. The keratome is again withdrawn and the other side of the incision is widened (c), thus completing the first plan of this two-plane incision. The anterior chamber is entered by placing the keratome at the initial stab wound, tilting the point down and advancing the blade.

The bottle can be slowly raised as position two is reached and by the time phacoemulsification begins the bottle can be restored to its normal height. Phacoemulsification is carried out in a routine manner. As with any surgery care is taken to avoid disrupting the iris, however, should this occur, the patient usually has no reaction. In a very rare case, vigorous stretching of the zonules may cause some patient discomfort. If this is of long duration or causes discomfort, small doses of IV supplemental anesthesia may be administered as well as additional drops of .5% tetracaine. This is a rare and transient situation.

Should iris prolapse occur during the procedure, the patient may experience a short

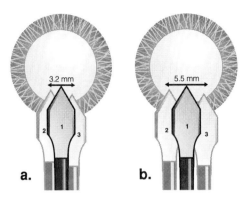

Figure 3.68a, b. IOL type determines where each of the three stages of wound construction will be placed. A 3.2-mm incision is used for foldable lenses (a), thus the three stabs are made closely together. A 5.5-mm incision is used for PMMA lenses (b) with the wound enlarged by placing the second and third stabs further away from the center of the initial incision.

burst of pain. This is generally due to stretching of the sphincter and it is very short lived. Care should be taken to reposit the iris gently so as not to exacerbate this situation. However, the iris appears to be less innervated by sensory fibers than previously thought.

Sphincterectomies may be routinely performed during phacoemulsification in eyes with small bound-down pupils. The patient generally experiences no discomfort from this. Likewise during trabeculectomies the peripheral iridectomy as well as the excision of trabecular tissue seems to cause no patient discomfort.

The irrigation/aspiration portion of the surgery is done with care to avoid the iris tissue. If at this or some other point during the procedure a posterior capsular tear is encountered, the procedure for continuing the operation is carried out in the same fashion as if the patient had a block. This can range from in the bag implantation to anterior vitrectomy and removal of nuclear remnants. In cases lasting up to 45 minutes, patients have been comfortable with additional topical anesthesia administered as required, usually every 15 minutes. It appears, at least in this time frame, the patient does not become refractory to the anesthetic. If suturing the implant through the sclera is attempted topical anesthesia is not a wise choice and should be augmented with peribulbar block because the area adjacent to the ciliary body is well supplied by sensory nerve fibers and the patient will be extremely uncomfortable.

In routine cases, implantation of either posterior or anterior chamber intraocular lenses including foldable lenses is done in the usual fashion. Wound closure with or without sutures is routine.

Iris suturing can be easily done under topical anesthesia. Astigmatic keratotomy performed during cataract extraction is made much easier with topical anesthesia as the patient fixates on the microscope light and both the visual and the horizontal and vertical axes are readily identifiable because the patient's globe is not distorted and fixation is available. These are two major advantages to this technique over using a block.

Injection of an agent for pupillary constriction (Miochol, Miostat) routinely causes the patient some minimal discomfort. Because Miochol is the weaker of the two solutions it is less likely to cause the ciliary spasm associated with transient pain. However, in a recent series of patients, surgery has been performed using Ocufen pre-operatively every 15 minutes beginning one hour prior to surgery. Epinephrine is removed from the

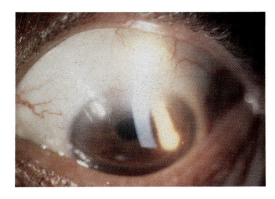

Figure 3.69. A quiet, clear eye immediately after surgery with a corneal incision.

irrigating solution and post-operatively Carbochol is used topically and in a corneal shield. These patients have satisfactorily miotic pupils one hour postoperatively. During surgery pupillary dilation has been adequate.

A corneal shield can also be used to deliver antibiotic-steroid in the post-operative period. The use of subconjuctival injections with topical anesthesia should be discouraged.

Post-Operative Procedure

Immediately post-operatively, the patient is asked to cover the non-operated eye and to glance around or read with generic reading glasses out of the operative eye. This sets the tone for very positive patient acceptance of the entire procedure. The patient is given two tablets of acetaminophine immediately post-operatively and is begun on antibiotic steroid combination drop immediately after surgery qid. A long acting beta blocker is given post-operatively the evening of surgery and the morning after surgery. In a series of 600 cases using this technique not one incidence of elevated intraocular pressure the day after surgery has been reported (Figure 3.69).

Summary

This technique is very useful in the vast majority of patients having cataract surgery as well as glaucoma procedures and refractive surgery. Good preparation is dependent on communication (vocal anesthesia) and the ability to judge patients. As with any other procedure, (phacoemulsification, extracapsular cataract extraction, etc.) the novice will gain more confidence with experience.

Editors' Comment

This presentation and that of Kershner and Williamson will all be discussed after the presentation of Williamson's technique.

ROBERT M. KERSHNER, MD
Orange Grove Eye Surgery Center, Tucson, AZ

No-Stitch Topical Anesthesia

Advances in the techniques of ECCE using phacoemulsification and small, self-sealing incisions have made local anesthesia preferable to general anesthesia for modern-day cataract surgery. The benefits of local injectable anesthetic include more rapid ambulation following cataract surgery, the ability to perform the procedure on an outpatient basis and general acceptance by patients.

Recently, peribulbar techniques of anesthesia have been described as substitutes for retrobulbar anesthesia. However, the risks of inadvertent ocular perforation, damage to the optic nerve, dural perforation, retrobulbar hemorrhage and death from orbital injection of anesthesia have also been described.

As cataract surgical techniques continue to improve with smaller self-sealing incisions, intercapsular phacoemulsification and IOL implantation through incisions of 3 mm or less, there has been a new opportunity created for shorter-acting and less-invasive anesthetic techniques. Richard A. Fichman, MD, first reported using topical anesthesia for cataract surgery. I have used topical anesthesia in 500 cataract cases.

Topical Technique

The patient is given one drop of Cyclomydril (cyclopentolate HCl, phenylephrine HCl) in the operative eye. An intravenous line is established. One drop of 0.5% Proparacaine (tetracaine HCl) is placed on the surface of the superior conjunctiva and the eyelids are scrubbed with Betadine. No ocular compression is performed. Sterile drapes are applied. Several drops of 0.5% Proparacaine are placed in the superior conjunctival cul-de-sac overlying the limbal peritomy site (Figure 3.70).

A wire eyelid speculum is placed, and the patient is asked to look down. No rectus bridle sutures are placed. The patient is told to expect a light from the microscope, to inform the surgeon of any discomfort, and to expect the sensation of the surgeon touching the eye.

Surgical Technique

A 4 mm limbal peritomy is created with a single snip of Westcott scissors at approximately 11:00, 4 mm from the vascular arcade. No cautery is employed. Using a diamond 2.85 mm keratome, a one-third-depth scleral groove is fashioned and the blade is used to tunnel through the sclera entering the eye anterior to Schwalbe's line at clear cornea (Figures 3.71 and 3.72). A one-step capsulorhexis is performed (Figures 3.73 and 3.74).

A double hydrodissection is performed with a curved Binkhorst-type cannula connected to a syringe filled with balanced salt solution, separating the lens cortex from the capsule.

Intercapsular phacoemulsification is performed and a viscoelastic is injected into the capsular bag (Figure 3.75). A one-piece silicone IOL is loaded in the injection cartridge and inserted through the scleral tunnel into the capsular bag (Figures 3.76).

The viscoelastic is removed, and the anterior chamber is inflated to normal pressure

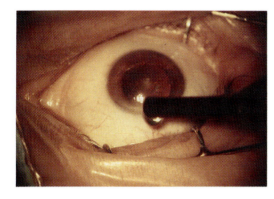

Figure 3.70. Topical anesthesia instilled in the superior conjunctival cul-de-sac prior to creating the incision.

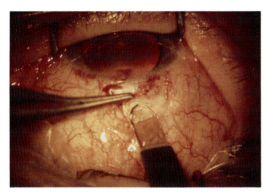

Figure 3.71.

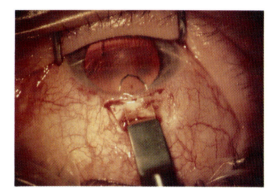

Figure 3.72.

Figures 3.71, 3.72. Creating the self-sealing tunnel with the one-step diamond 2.8 mm keratome.

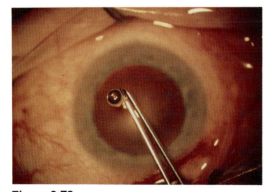

Figure 3.73.

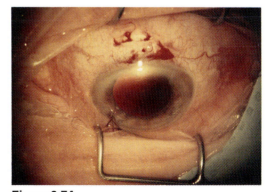

Figure 3.74.

Figures 3.73, 3.74. A 4 mm round capsulorhexis is made with the Kershner One-Step capsulorhexis forceps.

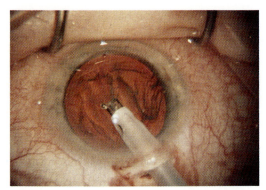

Figure 3.75. Intercapsular phacoemulsification performed through the central capsulorhexis entirely within the capsular bag.

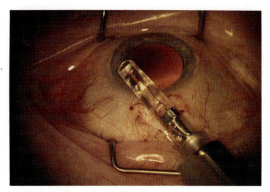

Figure 3.76 . The IOL placed in the injection cartridge.

with balanced salt solution. No ointment or eye patch is utilized. An injection of 0.3 cc of Ancef (cefazolin sodium) and Celestone (betamethasone sodium) is injected under the conjunctiva overlying the incision. The conjunctiva is neither cauterized nor sutured. The drapes are removed and the patient is questioned as to any discomfort, his ability to see with the operative eye and his experience during the surgery. The patient is then returned to a holding area prior to discharge.

Should any agitation or discomfort be noted by the patient, 10 mg/cc of Brevital is administered by the anesthesiologist 1 cc at a time, not to exceed a total volume of 4 to 6 cc as needed to induce relaxation and somnolence. In the first 500 patients, supplemental injection anesthesia was required 8% of the time.

Patients were asked a series of questions to evaluate their experience. In no case did a patient experience pain during the surgical procedure. Although patients were more aware of the surgeon touching the eyelids and the eye, and could see the light from the microscope, only 8% of patients found the experience disturbing enough to require supplemental intravenous sedation.

Technique Evolution

Over the past year, I have been modifying my anesthesia technique to find a way of anesthetizing the eye with rapid onset and short duration, allowing the patient to regain visual acuity as soon as possible following the surgery.

Initially, I used 3 cc of 2% Xylocaine in a modified peribulbar injection. This was quite effective in obtaining anesthesia as well as akinesia of the globe. Unfortunately, patients remained anesthetized for a minimum of four hours following surgery. They experienced double vision, blurred vision and inability to open or close the eyelid. A patient experiencing a retrobulbar hemorrhage from the injection might have to delay surgery and always experienced swelling and bruising of the eye and eyelids postoperatively.

Topical anesthesia provided complete analgesia during the surgery, which rapidly dissipated following surgery and in no way interfered with the patient's ability to blink, see or move the eye.

Akinesia of the globe, however, is not achieved with the procedure. Rectus bridle sutures were not used to avoid further discomfort, potential risk of globe perforation and increased risk of ptosis.

It is important to note that I firmly, yet gently, hold the eye with toothed forceps during the procedure until instruments are introduced into the eye. Once the conjunctiva is opened and the incision constructed, the capsulotomy forceps, phacoemulsification tip and lens implantation instrument allow control of the eye by an oarlock phenomenon (i.e., the eye cannot move out of position when the shaft of the instrument is in the incision tunnel).

Results

In the first 500 patients who underwent topical anesthesia without the use of a block, four experienced mild discomfort during the procedure. In no case did the patient experience pain while I was holding the eye or inserting instruments. As the eye is rotated inferiorly during the procedure, the microscope light is focused off the visual axis and did not appear uncomfortable for patients. Several were aware of changes in light and color as instruments were introduced into the eye, but none were disturbed by this experience.

Patients were most likely to be aware of the procedure during the limbal peritomy, grasping of the globe for incision construction and during IOL implantation. In no instance did the patient need supplemental injection anesthesia. However, intravenous Brevital was administered to a maximum of 40 mg (4 cc) if needed to aid in comfort and sedation.

During the surgical procedures, two observations were different from the usual procedure with injection anesthesia. First, without the retrobulbar fluid volume from injection and with normal muscle tension from the extraocular muscles, the globe rests more posteriorly in the orbit during surgery. The use of a wick was necessary during several procedures due to pooling of fluid. Second, the patient was able to aid in the surgery by looking in a desired direction, making exposure far more effective than during injection anesthesia when the globe was "frozen."

Summary

The major advantages of using topical anesthesia are decreased risk from needle injection. Patients prefer topical anesthesia with less intervention and medication. Patients appreciate the psychological advantage of being able to see immediately following the procedure. This is satisfying both to the patient and surgeon. In addition, the postoperative call on the afternoon of surgery allows the surgeon to assess the patient's vision rather than waiting until the following morning when a patch and/or anesthetic no longer interferes with vision. The patients are encouraged to use eye drops immediately following surgery and to take one or two acetaminophen tablets if needed.

Although topical anesthesia may not become the procedure of choice for every cataract surgeon, the benefits cannot be denied. As surgical techniques continue to improve, decreasing operative time with fewer intraoperative and postoperative risks, procedures that allow rapid return of vision by using topical anesthesia as an alternative to injection anesthesia demand careful consideration.

Editors' Comment

This presentation and that of Fichman and Williamson will all be discussed after the presentation of Williamson's technique.

CHARLES H. WILLIAMSON, MD
Williamson Eye Center, Baton Rouge, Louisiana

Clear Corneal Incision With Topical Anesthesia

The transition of intracapsular surgery to planned extracapsular and then phaco-emulsification has given surgeons greater control of the intraocular environment. Small incisions, scleral tunnel incisions, sutureless wounds, and now clear corneal incisions have reduced surgical trauma and sped healing and visual recovery. The safe implantation of an intraocular lens through small incisions became possible with the development of continuous circular capsulorhexis and foldable implants.

Delivering antibiotics through the infusion fluids seems to have reduced incidence of endophthalmitis in several large reported series. The advances in cataract surgery with less trauma, faster surgery, and greater control have allowed us to re-examine the use of topical anesthesia as the procedure of choice.

History

The Incas were responsible for the use of the world's first known topical anesthetic, cocaine. Tomas Morena y Maiz of Peru first suggested the medical use of cocaine as a topical anesthetic in 1868. Dr. Koller of Vienna and Dr. Sigmund Freud were the first to instill cocaine into the conjunctival sac for local anesthesia in 1884. Dr. Julius Hirschberg reported in 1910 that he had used 2% cocaine chloride solution for topical anesthesia in thousands of cataract procedures and "encountered only advantages, never a single disadvantage . . ."[76] In other reports, Drs. Jon Thorson, Arthur Jampolsky, and Alan Scott presented a paper in 1965 on topical anesthesia for strabismus surgery using Proparacaine HCL.[77] Dr. R. Smith of London performed extracapsular cataract extraction on 175 eyes of 165 patients from 1985 to 1988 under topical anesthesia with supplemental subconjunctival injection superiorly. Dr. Smith used Amethocaine 1% drops and 2% Xylocaine superiorly.[78] In 1991, Dr. Richard Fichman reported his cases of phacoemulsification under topical tetracaine.[79]

In 1992, I developed a technique using phacoemulsification through a stepped clear corneal wound under topical lidocaine in over 500 cases.[80]

Ideal Topical Anesthetic

The ideal topical anesthetic should be incapable of causing systemic toxicity and non-irritating; have low corneal toxicity, brief time of onset, and adequate duration of action.

Three topical anesthetics have been commonly used in eye surgery: tetracaine, proparacaine, and cocaine. Of these three, Proparacaine and cocaine have the greatest toxicity to the epithelium. Tetracaine, although much less toxic, does not produce adequate deep anesthesia and duration of action. Therefore, I believe the ideal topical ocular anesthetic is lidocaine.

The agent has been commonly used as a topical anesthetic for procedures in otolaryngology. I have used it in thousands of cases of radial keratotomy and 500 cases of phacoemulsification. It has the least toxicity on the epithelium, produces adequate deep anesthesia, and has a long duration of action.[81]

Advantages and Disadvantages of Topical Anesthesia

Topical anesthesia avoids potential complications of retrobulbar or peribulbar block which can include globe perforations, retrobulbar hemorrhage, optic nerve atrophy, retinal vascular occlusion, and ptosis. Systemic complications can include allergic reactions, systemic toxicity, intra-arterial injection, optic nerve sheath injection, and ocular cardiac reflex.

Risk on an individual basis is certainly small, but complications occur commonly. Although risks associated with peribulbar block are lower than those of retrobulbar block, numerous complications have still been reported.[82] With the use of topical anesthesia these significant complications can be avoided. All other major complications related to cataract surgery are on the decline, except those associated with regional block anesthesia.

The use of topical anesthesia obviates any medical contraindications to cataract surgery. In regional block anesthesia it is common to significantly sedate patients in combination with the block. This level of sedation can cause respiratory compromise. Many systemic complications are possible with regional block anesthesia. Topical anesthesia gives an extra margin of safety in the medically compromised patient.

Topical anesthesia allows for the fastest visual rehabilitation in history. Patients may go home without a patch and see clearly immediately after the surgery. In my practice some patients have achieved 20/20 uncorrected vision just 30 minutes after phacoemulsification with clear corneal incisions under topical Lidocaine.

The disadvantages of topical anesthesia include potential eye movement during phacoemulsification and patient anxiety.

A common factor mentioned in most papers on topical anesthesia for the last 100 years is that eye movement has always been easily controlled and has not been a problem during surgery in thousands of patients. It is sometimes helpful that the patient can move his eyes to a more advantageous position on command.

Patient anxiety can usually be easily controlled with communication. Assuring the patient that there will be no pain and reporting the progress of the procedure will usually calm any fear or trepidation. Certainly mild IV sedation can be used as an adjunct if needed.

Patient Selection

Patients who are unable to cooperate or follow instructions include those with such conditions as dementia, deafness, or inability to communicate are contraindicated for topical anesthesia and would most likely do better under regional block anesthesia with IV sedation. Surgery on an inflamed eye should be performed under retrobulbar block. Cataract surgery in children should be performed under general anesthesia.

Relative contraindications may be a small pupil in which there may be significant iris manipulation or cases of planned extracapsular surgery in which very large scleral incisions are performed. However, it is certainly possible to perform phacoemulsification through pupils as small as 3 to 4 mm without significant manipulation. Planned extracapsular cataract surgery can be performed under topical anesthesia with adjunct use of a subconjunctival limbal injection of Xylocaine.

Technique

Two drops of 0.5% tetracaine are usually instilled into the operative eye prior to dilation. Tetracaine is used because it is readily available, prevents the stinging from the dilating drops, and is placed into the eye quite some time before surgery is scheduled to occur (Figure 3.78). A routine dilation regimen with mydriatics with or without nonsteroidal anti-inflammatory agents may be used.

Individual TB syringes are filled with 4% lidocaine from a 50 cc bottle (Figure 3.79). These are drawn up by the nurse and are labeled for each patient. The needle is then removed and the syringe is capped to serve as an individual medicine dropper (Figure 3.80). Two sets of topical 4% lidocaine, four drops every five to 10 minutes is begun before entering the operating room. A heparin lock is placed in the hand opposite the operative eye (Figure 3.81).

As soon as the patient enters the operating room and is positioned, four more drops of topical 4% lidocaine are instilled into the operative eye. Routine cataract prep consists of two drops of 5% Betadine solution in the conjunctival sac and a Betadine scrub of the periocular area. The patient is draped and the lid speculum is inserted just before the surgeon arrives.

The standby supplies in the operating room include 1% Xylocaine with syringes and needles for sterile peribulbar or subconjunctival block if needed. Intravenous sedation with Versed (1 mg) or Brevital (15-20 mg) is also be available in the operating room if the surgeon believes this is necessary to relieve patient anxiety. Sterile Tetracaine should be available if needed.

It is important to never oversedate a patient under topical anesthesia because they will be unable to cooperate with the surgeon's instructions.

Patients who undergo tunnel incision surgery and phacoemulsification from the traditional superior approach may have better eye position with a bridle suture in place. If the use of a bridle suture is needed, then it is helpful to infiltrate the superior conjunctiva with 1% Xylocaine just prior to passing the bridle suture.

Surgical Technique

It is important to adhere to rigid patient selection and a strict preoperative regimen in early cases. This would include a well dilated pupil to prevent excessive iris manipulation. Orbital decompression devices such as the Honan balloon® or Super Pinky® should be avoided because they are uncomfortable and unnecessary since there is no solution in the orbit to cause external pressure. I have found that all the eyes under topical anesthesia are quite soft and have absolutely no problems from posterior pressure.

In my opinion the injection of several milliliters of anesthetic in the orbital space causes many of the posterior pressure problems in intraocular surgery. The retrobulbar injection itself can also cause a dull postoperative orbital pain.

Since the patient's eyes are anesthetized in the preoperative area, nurses request that patients keep the eyes closed to prevent corneal exposure and drying of the cornea before surgery.

If the patient arrives on the operative table with a poorly dilated pupil, more time can be allowed for further dilation and epinephrine may be used in an irrigating solution. With very small pupils (less than 3 mm), it may be advisable to use 1% Xylocaine injected subconjunctivally as an adjunct to the procedure before draping.

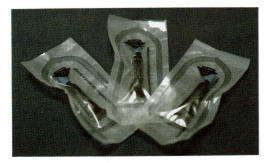

Figure 3.78. Tetracaine drops instilled preoperatively.

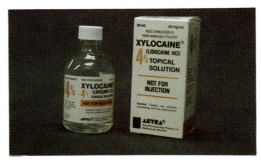

Figure 3.79. 50 cc bottle of 4% topical lidocaine.

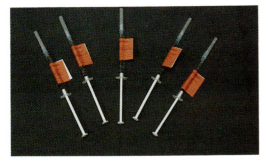

Figure 3.80. Individual syringes filled with 4% topical lidocaine and labeled.

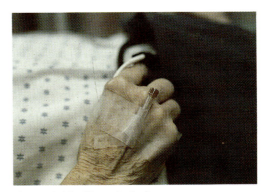

Figure 3.81. Heparin lock.

There is a learning curve associated in draping the lids under topical anesthesia. The patient is asked to look straight ahead and the wooden ends of cotton tipped applicators are used to retract the lids. A non-fenestrated plastic drape with adhesive is then placed on the eye so that the lashes are pressed back against the upper and lower lids. The drape is then carefully cut to avoid bringing the lateral edge of the drape incision past the lateral canthal angle.

A bladed lid speculum is then inserted. This is usually adequate to prevent reflex closure of the eyelids during surgery and to keep the lashes out of the surgical field. The corner of an unfolded 3 X 3 sponge is inserted into the cul-de-sac of the lateral canthal angle. This serves as a wick for fluid collecting temporally and also covers an area in which the lashes have a tendency to be more exposed when performing the surgery from a temporal approach.

Intraoperative Eye Position

If the patient has poor eye position during surgery, it is important to communicate with the patient so that he or she may assist in achieving the proper eye position. Performing surgery from a temporal approach is usually more easily done because the patient is asked to fixate straight ahead on the light of the operating microscope. Since patients are usually very comfortable with looking straight ahead, the eyes seem to rarely move. This makes the temporal surgical approach an excellent choice for this type of anesthesia. A temporal surgical approach is mandatory in clear corneal incisions.

If the surgery is performed with the traditional scleral tunnel from above, the patient usually must look down if no bridle suture is used. Patients may have difficulty maintaining this eye position throughout the surgery making a bridle suture necessary. Adjunctive subconjunctival infiltration with Xylocaine may be needed in these cases. When performing phacoemulsification, there is greater control once the instruments are in the eye and "oarlocked" in the tunnel to provide fixation.

Inadequate Anesthesia

The patient should be entirely comfortable after the initial lidocaine drops. I have found very few cases in which the patient experienced pain either during or after the surgery. If the patient does have a burning sensation at the beginning or during the procedure, additional anesthetic drops may be required. If after the initial drops in the preoperative area, the patient feels any stinging sensation from the drops delivered in the operating room prior to surgery, then it may be necessary to check the effectiveness of the lidocaine.

Four percent lidocaine seems to be most effective if used during the first week after opening the bottle. Very rarely, a bad lot may be distributed. To test for this, the surgeon may place a few drops of the topical anesthetic on the tip of his or her tongue. There should be an immediate onset of deep anesthesia. (The tongue test will convince the surgeon of the effectiveness of topical lidocaine on mucous membranes.)

Occasionally, patients may experience a dull headache or pressure type discomfort caused by over-expansion of the anterior chamber. It is important to maintain normal fluidic and hydraulic control of the anterior chamber. In clear corneal tunnel incisions with phaco. The bottle is raised slightly higher than normal. There are some positive pressure hydraulic control systems available on a number of phaco units which seem to keep a more quiet and stable anterior chamber. These are presently being studied and may have a place with the use of topical anesthesia. Mild sedation may also be helpful (never oversedate).

Any sudden sharp pain is usually transient and only caused by significant iris trauma. Indeed, even an iridectomy may be performed with only mild discomfort.

Patient Anxiety

I have found the most useful tool to relieve patient anxiety is simply communication with the patient. Certainly, very mild IV sedation with Brevital (15 to 20 mg) or Versed (1 mg) is an option and may be used routinely if the surgeon prefers. However, it is very important to never oversedate the patient. Oversedated patients are unable to cooperate properly during the surgery.

Phacoemulsification is clearly the procedure of choice in using topical anesthesia. Smaller wounds and less trauma allow greater patient comfort. There is also greater control of the eye when the instruments are in the wounds which provides excellent fixation. While planned extracapsular procedures can be performed under topical anesthesia, it usually advisable to use adjunctive subconjunctival Xylocaine (1 to 2 cc) superiorly.

Since less trauma is certainly more desirable for the patient under topical anesthesia, the fewer sutures needed the better. While "sutureless" self-sealing corneal wounds are ideal for topical anesthesia, sutures can be used quite easily with little discomfort.

Incisions Under Topical Anesthesia

The ideal surgery for topical anesthesia is a clear corneal incision performed from a temporal approach, first introduced by Dr. I. Howard Fine in April 1992. I subsequently developed a technique of stepped clear corneal tunnel incision performed under topical lidocaine. A 3.5 mm half thickness corneal groove is made with a special diamond blade step-knife (Figures 3.82 and 3.83).

This diamond keratome was designed to fashion a rhomboid-shaped, 2-mm long corneal tunnel from the temporal approach (3.2 mm internal opening and 3.5 mm external opening). After continuous circular capsulorhexis, bi-manual phacoemulsification is performed. After irrigation and aspiration, viscoelastic is used to inflate the capsular bag.

A Staar Model AA4203 elastic lens is introduced through the tunnel and into the capsular bag using the Microstaar injector (Figure 3.84). This procedure is performed without sutures and the internal corneal valve mechanism provides a water tight wound. This surgery should always be performed temporally as this position avoids the conjunctival overhang found superiorly and also places the wound at the furthest position from the visual axis. Temporal placement of the corneal tunnel allows for faster postop

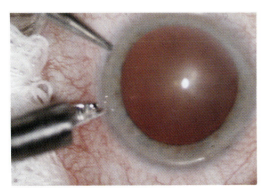

Figure 3.82. Corneal groove is fashioned.

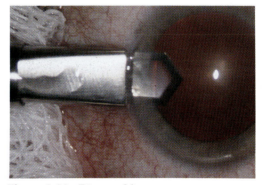

Figure 3.83. Diamond keratome entry.

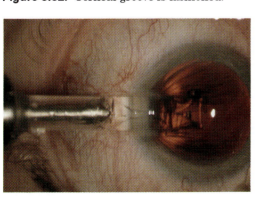

Figure 3.84. Injection of Staar AA4203 elastic lens with Microstaar injector.

visual recovery as well as minimal induced astigmatism in the visual axis secondary to corneal edema in the area of the tunnel.

Scleral tunnel incisions may be performed under topical anesthesia, but are best performed from the temporal approach. Although less desirable than clear corneal incisions, the temporal approach in scleral tunnel incisions still allows excellent surgical exposure even in the most deep set eyes and there is never a need for a bridle suture to be performed. The instruments in the wound (especially using the bimanual technique) are able to fixate the eye quite readily and counteract any natural Bell's phenomenon which may occur if the patient tries to close the eye.

A scleral tunnel from the superior approach may also be performed under topical anesthesia but has the disadvantage of having to ask the patient to look down constantly unless a bridle suture is used. If a bridle suture is performed, it is then best to use adjunctive subconjunctival 1% Xylocaine (1 to 2 cc) superiorly.

Post-operative Care

Topical antibiotic-steroid drops are instilled in the operative eye before the patient leaves the operating room. The lid is taped for 20 to 30 minutes while the patient is in the postoperative area to avoid any corneal exposure which may occur while the anesthesia is still in effect.

When the patient is discharged from the postoperative area, the tape is removed and the patient may start a routine regimen of postoperative antibiotic-steroid drops immediately. If the patient feels any mild transient burning sensation, this is easily treated with lubricant drops. I have found the patients report very little discomfort.

When using a clear corneal incision, I prefer to put a disposable contact lens on the eye as a bandage to cover the eye and protect the wound from potential contamination since the eye is not patched. My patients seem much more comfortable postoperatively than when I was using regional block anesthesia.

Complications

There are few complications with topical anesthesia. Systemic reactions are virtually unheard of when using topical lidocaine in the prescribed doses and have not occurred in any of my cases. While a local allergic reaction is possible, it would be immediately apparent with hyperemia, stinging, and itching as well as chemosis of the conjunctiva. It is also possible for delayed hypersensitivity to occur as well. I have never encountered a case of local allergic reaction using topical lidocaine.

Summary

The rediscovery of topical anesthesia for routine cataract surgery has been made possible through evolution in surgical techniques which provide more control during surgery with less trauma and smaller wounds. It seems that a clear corneal incision technique with phacoemulsification from the temporal approach is the ideal procedure performed under topical anesthesia.

I have found lidocaine to be the best agent for use as a topical anesthetic. Topical anesthesia completely eliminates the potential complication of blindness from retrobulbar or peribulbar block. It obviates medical contraindications to cataract surgery, provides better patient comfort, fewer surgical complications, reduced costs, and instantaneous visual rehabilitation.

Editors' Comment

As minimally invasive cataract and glaucoma surgery continue to evolve many more procedures may be done expertly with topical anesthesia; it will then become the responsibility of the surgeon to devote the time to the preoperative selection of patients and their education so that regional anesthesia and general anesthesia are no longer necessary, except for selected patients. Thus selection of patients will become very critical for the technique to produce reliable results.

All three authors mention the sensitivity of the zonules and ciliary body to painful stimuli and the relative lack of pain response in the central iris. At what concentration can local anesthetics be safely irrigated in the anterior chamber to reduce iris, zonule, and ciliary body pain?

We look forward to statistical analysis of controlled studies of excellent surgical results and increased anesthesia safety. However, enthusiastic patients will not be the measure of success—rather prevention of unhappy anesthetic and poor visual results.

One of the editors (JPG) has now used the technique very successfully with 150 patients and their enthusiasm and excellent surgical results are incentive to a much more widespread use of the technique for selected patients.

Conclusions

Injection Anesthesia

Skill at avoiding delicate structures is 99% anatomical insight and 1% feedback of information from the needle and patient. Skill in using the feedback from the needle and patient and applying it to anatomical insight is very important and comes with experience. Models can be developed which will let the beginner appreciate those facts faster. However, the main contribution is anatomical insight, and that comes only from studying 3-D models and developing 3-D skill with needles.

This chapter is written as an incentive to provide better training programs for residents or anesthesia providers to learn better and safer orbital anesthesia and to their teachers—who will assume the legal and ethical responsibilities of safer and better anesthesia for patients.

Orbital/ocular anesthesia terminology needs to be clarified in keeping with Koornneef's anatomical findings of the spatial structure of the orbit. In particular, he has demonstrated that although there are discrete intermuscular septa between the anterior portions of the tendons of the four rectus muscles, these interrectus muscle septa cease to exist as the posterior surface of the globe is reached—a fact recognized by Atkinson.[4,13-21]

With the various modifications in anesthesia technique implemented to increase safety or efficacy the distinctions among "orbital," "peribulbar," "periocular," and "retrobulbar" injections and the resultant anesthesia have become blurred; we are now in a situation where the injection locus may be the same for techniques but different names are applied to imply effectiveness or safety.

Knowledge of anatomy, geometry, and technical skill increase efficacy. Knowledge of anatomy and skill at avoiding delicate structures, not better names, increases safety.

Injuries are inadvertent; diagnosis and treatment along optimum guidelines are essential to prove absence of negligence.

Topical Anesthesia

"First, do no harm," the primary maxim in medicine, should be the overriding concern when any new technique or procedure is developed, and that certainly holds true for topical ocular anesthesia.

As in any surgical procedure, when using topical anesthesia there are strict guidelines to which ophthalmologists must adhere to achieve good results safely. That regimen includes patient selection criteria, the knowledge of when to convert to regional block anesthesia during a complicated case, and how to control surgery and monitor patient reaction.

Suitable topical patients should be routine cataract surgery candidates who are alert and able to follow directions and control their movements. Patients who are deaf, demented, photophobic, or cannot communicate are contraindicated for topical anesthesia, as are children. Surgery on inflamed eyes should be done under retrobulbar block. Likewise, patients with small pupils who may need significant iris manipulations or those who need large scleral incisions may be contraindicated for topical anesthesia.

The ability to communicate well with patients, confidence in the technique, and expertise in cataract surgery, especially phacoemulsification, are prerequisites for good outcomes. Additionally, it is necessary that surgeons understand the effects of oral or intravenous sedation on the patient and when to convert to regional block anesthesia.

And while topical anesthesia may not become the procedure of choice for every cataract surgeon in every case, its proponents cite the elimination of potential blindness from retro- or peribulbar block, fewer surgical complications, less intervention and medication, and the ability to see well almost immediately post-operatively as self-evident benefits.

References

1. Van Lint A. Paralysie palpébrale temporarie provoquée dans l'opération de la cataract. Ann Ocul (Paris) 151:420;1914.
2. Wright RE. Blocking of the main trunk of the facial nerve in surgery. Arch Ophthalmol 55:55-6;1926.
3. O'Brien CS. Akinesis during cataract extraction. Arch Ophthalmol 1:447-9;1929.
4. Atkinson WS. Local anesthesia in ophthalmology. Tr Am Ophth Soc 32:399-451;1934.
5. Seidel E. Ueber eine modifikation der Seigristschen methode der lokal anesthesie bei exenteratio und enuclatio bulbi. Kleinische Manatsble f Augenh 49:329;1911.
6. Siegrist A. Lokalanästhesie bei exentertio und enucleatio bulbi. Klin Monatsbl f Augenh 45:106-9;1907.
7. Duverger. L'anesthésie locale en ophtalmologie. Masson et CM^{ie}, Paris, 1920.
8. Knapp H. On cocaine and its use in ophthalmic and general surgery. Arch Ophthalmol 13:402;1884.
9. Lowenstein A. Ueber regionare anasthesie in der orbita. Klin Monatsb f Augenh 592-601;1908.
10. Gifford SR. The prevention of complications in the cataract operation. Illinois Medical Journal 68:243-4;1935.
11. Greenwood A, Grossman HP. Analysis of 1,343 intracapsular cataract extractions by 48 operators following the Verhoett method. Trans Am Ophtal Soc 33:353-61;1935.
12. de Grosz E. L'extraction de la cataract d'après 15,000 opérations. Arch d'Opht 53:161-5;1936.
13. Atkinson WS. Retrobulbar injection of anesthetic within the muscular cone. Arch Ophth 16:494-503;1936.
14. Atkinson WS. Local anesthesia in ophthalmology. Arch Ophthalmol 30:777-80;1943.
15. Atkinson WS. Local anesthesia in ophthalmology. Am J Ophthalmol 31:1607-18;1948.
16. Atkinson WS. Use of hyaluronidase with local anesthesia in ophthalmology. Arch Ophthalmol 42:628-

33;1949.

17. Atkinson WS. Anesthesia in Ophthalmology, First Edition. Charles C. Thomas, Springfield, 1955.

18. Atkinson WS. Observation of anesthesia for ocular surgery. Trans Amer Acad Ophthalmol & Otolaryngol 60:376-80;1956.

19. Atkinson WS. Ophthalmic anesthesia: the development of ophthalmic anesthesia. Am J Ophthalmol 51:1-14;1961.

20. Atkinson WS. Larger volume retrobulbar injections. Am J Ophthalmol 57:328;1964.

21. Atkinson WS. Anesthesia in Ophthalmology, Second Edition. Charles C. Thomas, Springfield, 1965.

22. Gifford H Jr. Motory block of extraocular muscles by deep orbital injection. Arch Ophthalmol 41:5-19;1949.

22b. Gifford H Jr. Discussion. Tr Amer Acad Opthalmol & Otolaryngol 363-5;May/June 1954.

23. Kirsch RE. Further studies on the use of digital pressure in cataract surgery. Arch Ophthalmol 58:641-4;1957.

24. Scheie HG, Ellis RA, et al. Long-lasting local anesthetic agents in ophthalmic surgery. Arch Ophthalmol 53:177-90;1955.

25. Lichter P. The relative value of quality care. Ophthalmology 98:1151-2;1991.

26. Gills JP, Loyd TL. A technique of retrobulbar block with paralysis of orbicularis oculi. Am Intra-ocular Implant Soc J 9:339;1983.

27. Johnson DE, Gills JP. Advanced ophthalmic anesthesia. Current Therapy in Ophthalmic Surgery. Ed. Spaeth AL, Katz LJ, Parker KW. BC Decker, Inc., Toronto, 1989. pp 1-5.

28. Davis DB II, Mandel MR. Posterior peribulbar anesthesia: An alternative to retrobulbar anesthesia. J Cataract Refract Surg 12:182-4;1986.

29. Davis DB II, Mandel MR. Peribulbar anesthesia (letter). J Cataract Refract Surg 16:527-8;1990.

30. Bloomberg L. Administration of periocular anesthesia. J Cataract Refract Surg 12:677-9;1986.

31. Bloomberg L. Anterior peribulbar anesthesia: Five years experience. J Cataract Refract Surg 17:508-11;1991.

32. Wang HS. Peribulbar anesthesia for ophthalmic procedures. J Cataract Refract Surg 14:441-3;1988.

33. Dixon C. The Sprotte, Whitacre, and Quincke spinal needles. Anesthesiology Review 18:42-7;Sept/Oct 1991.

34a. Braun H. Local Anesthesia. Translated and edited by Harris ML. Loa & Febiger, Philadelphia, 1924. p 180.

34b. ibid, pp 218-9. 35. McMahon D. Managing regional anesthesia equipment. Problems in Anesthesia 1:592-601;1987.

36. Grajewski A, Fernandez O, Keilson L, Galindo A. Importance of needle tip in retro-peribulbar anesthesia. To be published in Ophthalmology.

37. Allen CW. Local and Regional Anesthesia, Second Edition. WB Saunders Company, 1918. p 647.

38. Vorosmarthy D. Oculopression: types and methods of application, possibilities of utilization. Bibliotheca Ophthalmologica 69:42-99;1966.

39. Gills JP. Constant mild compression of the eye to produce hypotension. Am Intra-ocular Implant Soc J 5:52-3;1979.

40. McDonneel P, Quigley H, et al. The honan intraocular pressure reducer. Arch Ophthalmol 103:422-5;1985.

41. Thornton SP. Consultation Section. Ed. Shepard DD. J Cataract Refract Surg 12:425;1986.

42. Palay D, Stulting R. The effect of external ocular compression on intra-ocular pressure following retrobulbar anesthesia. Ophthalmic Surg 21:503-7;1990.

43. Ropo A, Ruusuvaara P, et al. Effect of ocular compression (Autopressor) on intraocular pressure in periocular anesthesia. Acta Ophthalmol Copenh 68:227-9;1990.

44. Zable RW, Clarke WN, et al. Intraocular pressure reduction prior to retrobulbar injection of anesthetic. Ophthalmic Surg 19:868-71;1988.

45. Otto AJ, Spekreijse H. Volume discrepancies in the orbit and the effect on the intra-orbital pressure: an experimental study in the monkey. Orbit 8:233-44;1989.

46. Bloomberg L. Periocular method of anesthesia administration called safe, easy. Ophthalmology Times 54-5;Feb 1986.

47. Cowley M, Campochiaro PA, et al. Retinal vascular occlusion without retrobulbar or optic nerve sheath hemorrhage after retrobulbar injection of lidocaine. Ophthalmic Surg 19:859-61;1988.

48. Brod RD. Transient central retinal artery occlusion and central lateral amaurosis after retrobulbar anesthetic injection. Ophthalmic Surg 20:643-5;1989.

49. Jindra L. Blindness following retrobulbar anesthesia for astigmatic keratotomy. Ophthalmic Surg 20:433-5;1989.

50. Davis II DB, Mandel MR. Peribulbar anesthesia, a review of technique and complications. Ophthalmology Clinics of North America 3:101-9;March 1990.

51. Weiss J, Deichman C. A comparison of retrobulbar and periocular anesthesia for cataract surgery. Arch Ophthalmol 107:96-8;1989.
52. Adriani J. Labat's Regional Anesthesia. Warren H. Green, Inc., St. Louis, 1985.
53a. Pitkin GP. Conduction Anesthesia. Ed. Southworth JL, Hingson RA. JB Lippincott Co., Philadelphia, 1946. pp 333-8.
53b. ibid, pp 336.
54. Unsold R, Stanley J, Degroot J. The CT topography of retrobulbar anesthesia. Albrecht von Graefes Arch Klin Ophthalmol 217:125-36;1981.
55. Grizzard WS. Ophthalmic anesthesia. Ophthalmology Annual. Ed. Reinecke RD. Raven Press, New York, 1989.
56. Hamilton RC, Gimbel HV, Strunin L. Regional anaesthesia for 12,000 cataract extraction and intraocular lens implantation procedures. Can J Anaesth 35:615-23;1988.
57. Martin S, Baker S, Muenzler W. Retrobulbar anesthesia and orbicularis akinesia. Ophthalmic Surg 17:232-33;1986.
58. Morgan CM, Schatz H, et al. Ocular complications associated with retrobulbar injections. Ophthalmology 95:660-5;1988.
59. Grizzard WS, Kirk N, et al. Perforating ocular injuries caused by anesthesia personnel. Ophthalmology 98:1011-6;1991.
60. Hamilton RC. Non-ophthalmologists and orbital regional anesthesia (letter). Ophthalmology 99:169-70;1992.
61. Katsev DA, Drews RC, Rose BT. An anatomic study of retrobulbar needle path length. Ophthalmology 96:1221-4;1989.
62. Buttery R, Wise G. Conal anesthesia: A new approach to retrobulbar anaesthesia. Australian and New Zealand J Ophthalmol 17:63-9;1989.
63. Rosenblatt RM, May DR, Barsoumian K. Cardiopulmonary arrest after retrobulbar block. Am J Ophthalmol 90:425-7;1980.
64. Smith JL. Retrobulbar marcaine can cause respiratory arrest. J Clin Neuro-ophthalmol 1:171-2;1981.
65. Beltranena HP, Vega MJ, et al. Complications of retrobulbar marcaine injection. J Clin Neuro-ophthalmol 2:159-61;1982.
66. Zaturansky MD, Hyam SS. Perforation of the globe during the injection of local anesthesia. Opthalmic Surg 18:585-8;1987.
67. Juei-Ling Chang, Gonzalez-Abola E, et al. Brain stem anesthesia following retrobulbar block (letter). Anesthesiology 61:798-90;1984.
68. Pautler S, Grizzard WS. Blindness from retrobulbar injection into the optic nerve. Ophthalmic Surg 17:334-7;1986.
69. Wittpenn JR, Rapoza P, et al. Respiratory arrest following retrobulbar anesthesia. Ophthalmology 93:867-70;1986.
70. Brookshire G, Gleitsmann K, Schenk E. Life-threatening complication of retrobulbar block: A hypothesis. Ophthalmology 93:1476-8;1986.
71. Kimble JA, Morris RE, et al. Globe perforation from peribulbar injection. Arch Ophthalmol 105:749;1987.
72. Gills JP. Anesthesia for cataract extraction. J Cataract Refract Surg 12:182-5;1986.
73. Mastel D. Needle quality. Ocular Surgery News 33:Feb 1 1988.
74. Kimbrough RG, Stewart RH, Okereke PC. A modified Gill's block and its effectiveness for lid akinesia. Ophthalmic Surg 18:14-7;1987.
75. Hustead RF. Patent #5, 134, 991.
76. Hirschberg J. History of Ophthalmology 284;1910.
77. Thorson J, Jampolsky A, Scott A. Topical Anesthesia for Strabismus Surgery. Trans Am Acd Ophthmol & Otol 70:968-972;1966.
78. Smith R. Cataract Extraction Without Retrobulbar Injection. Brit J Ophthalmol April:205-107;1990.
79. Fichman R. American Society of Cataract and Refractive Surgery Meeting-April 1992.
80. Williamson CH. Cataract Keratotomy with Topical Anesthesia. Ocular Sur News Vol 10 No 15:44; 1992.
81. Marr WG, Wood R, Senterfit L, Sigelman S. Effect of Topical Anesthesia on Regeneration of Corneal Epithelium. Am J Ophthalmol 43:606-610;1957.
82. Zahl K, Meltzer MA. The Complications of Regional Anesthesia in Ophthalmology Clinics of North America. March:111-123;1990.

Four

Robert C. Hamilton, MB, BCh
W. Sanderson Grizzard, MD

COMPLICATIONS

Introduction

The complications of regional anesthesia for ophthalmology may be systemic, or confined to the orbit and its contents, and may be acute in onset or delayed. They range from minor effects to the death of the patient. This chapter covers various complications, their incidence as reported in the literature, discussions regarding clinical management, and how best to avoid them. Some are directly related to the local anesthetic drugs and administration techniques, while other are surgical in nature, occurring only after operative intervention.

In many centers patients routinely receive sedative or narcotic drugs, often intravenously, to facilitate anesthetic techniques. By employing low stimulus methods, sedative drugs may not be necessary or only used in low dosage when necessary. Side effects and complications related to the use and misuse of sedative drugs are thus minimized.[1,2] Intravenous sedative medication may occasionally be required for markedly anxious patients.

Excellent surgical outcome is strongly influenced by good anesthesia. The most appropriate management of an inadequate anesthetic block is supplemental injection of further local anesthetic agent rather than the suppression of reactivity with systemic medication.

Selection of Patients

Patient cooperation is a prerequisite for ophthalmic regional anesthesia. It is wise to decide early on an appropriate alternative if there is doubt. General anesthesia is the preferred method for procedures lasting more than 90 minutes. Patients with dementia, mental retardation, uncontrollable cough or marked head tremor may be poor candidates for regional anesthesia. Pre-teens are better served by general anesthesia.

Personal confidence is acquired with repeated use of regional anesthesia technique,[3] and patients respond positively to that increased confidence. They are more stable and reassured, and less dependent on premedicant drugs.[4] Simple measures like the positioning arthritic patients for maximum comfort, prewarming local anesthetics to near body temperature,[5] the use of topical anesthetic drops prior to transconjunctival injections, and having a member of the team hold the patient's hand throughout the operative procedure are beneficial.[6]

Prologue

The eye is naturally well protected within the orbit from injury (Figure 4.1). However, it is not surprising that medical intervention with needles can result in complications. The anatomy has been extensively reviewed in Chapter One. To achieve the desired goals of globe and adnexal anesthesia and akinesia with concurrent hypotony, a two injection method became the traditionally accepted technique, combining the deposition of a small volume of local anesthetic at the apex of the orbit with a block of the seventh nerve at some point along its extracranial path.[7-12]

The safety of injecting a small volume of anesthetic at the apex has been challenged in the past decade because of damage to structures behind the eye with retrobulbar and posterior peribulbar needles. The need for separate blocking of the seventh nerve has been questioned because akinesia of the orbicularis, adequate for cataract surgery at least, is associated with larger volume injections in the anterior orbit. Avoiding a seventh nerve block frees the patient of that painful maneuver and the risks of anatomical complications.

Complications: Prevention, Assessment, and Treatment

Percutaneous Seventh Nerve Block Complications

Several articles report complications with blocking of the main trunk of the facial nerve after its exit from the stylomastoid foramen.[13-15] Swallowing difficulty and respiratory obstruction related to unilateral vagus, glossopharyngeal and spinal accessory blockade were noted. Needles longer than advocated by Nadbath and Rehman had been used and hyaluronidase, not part of the classical block,[9] had often been used. Five cases of facial nerve paralysis caused by local anesthetic blocks in four patients with injection of the main trunk[12] and in one blocked by the O'Brien method[3] anterior to the tragus of the ear[16] have been reported.

Superb anesthesia along with excellent periorbital muscle akinesia may be obtained without a separate percutaneous seventh nerve blockade due to improved anesthetic agents and the introduction of orbital decompression devices that allow the injection of larger volumes of local anesthetics. Because larger volumes of anesthetic are injected in the orbit, it is all the more important that mechanisms causing complications from larger injections be fully understood.

Brainstem Anesthesia[17]

In the late 1960s some unexpected sequelae of radiologic techniques were reported including the demonstration radiographically of communication from the subdural space

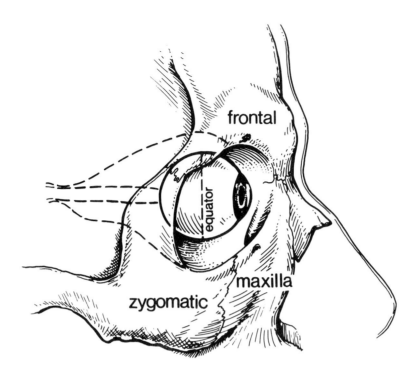

Figure 4.1 The equator of the eye is generally at, or slightly anterior to the lateral orbital rim. The position of the eye is variable and must be assessed in each patient prior to injection. The eye is generally closer to the roof of the orbit than the floor, and the frontal bone overhangs the eye making the inferotemporal approach the most open access to the retrobulbar space. (Reproduced with permission from WS Grizzard and Raven Press)

of the optic nerve to the chiasm and into the subarachnoid space surrounding the pons and midbrain.[18,19] Cadaver experiments confirmed these findings.[20,21] With traditional techniques, using 22 and 23 gauge dull needles the optic nerve sheath may not have been easily penetrated. The more common occurrence of brainstem anesthesia in the past decade may be related to use of sharp disposable needles which can more easily engage the sheath, although the physicochemical characteristics of bupivacaine plays a significant role, as does the use of larger volumes of anesthetic injection.

Serious central nervous system depression following retrobulbar block was reported sporadically between 1886 and 1980, but became epidemic in 1980.[22-27] The administered dose was insufficient to explain the clinical picture of unconsciousness and apnea based on systemic drug levels, and the time sequence did not usually support an intra-arterial injection as the explanation[28] (except in one case[4]). An allergic mechanism did not fit, as patients experiencing the problem often had an uncomplicated operation on the contralateral eye using an identical technique.[29]

Although there was knowledge of the meningeal pathway from the optic nerve to the midbrain, it was not until the mid-1980s that publications favored that mechanism as being the cause. Kobet reported a case of brainstem anesthesia following retrobulbar block in which a higher level of lidocaine was found in lumbar cerebrospinal fluid than could be accounted for from systemic distribution.[30] In several larger reported series it became clear that the effect of spread of local anesthetic in the central nervous system during retrobulbar block depends on the amount of drug entering and the specific area to which it spreads.[29,31-35] An incidence as high as 0.79% is stated in one paper[35] but more commonly is reported as one case per 350 to 500 patients.[29,31,32,34,36] Hustead has not seen one in 20,000 cases.

From these papers a clear pattern of local anesthetic effects can be listed. Typically the patient first describes symptoms of drowsiness with onset at about two minutes after the orbital injection. Frequently the zenith culminating in apnea is not reached until 10 to 20 minutes and resolves over two to three hours.

As brainstem anesthesia is always a potential complication, patients should not be draped for surgery until 15 minutes after block completion, otherwise identification and corrective treatment may be dangerously delayed. An essential prerequisite in all locations where regional ocular anesthesia is performed is the ability to provide pulmonary support and nearby access to cardiopulmonary resuscitation equipment.[24,29,30,37-39] Surgery is often possible immediately following recovery from the complication.

Ophthalmologists most commonly administer the local anesthetic for eye surgery; however, with the increasing popularity of fast turnover day-case cataract surgery, anesthesia personnel increasingly administer regional anesthesia for eye surgery. This frees up the ophthalmologist in a busy practice to use time more efficiently, and the patient has the advantage of undivided and continuing attention. More than half of the large volume practices delegate the administration of blocks to anesthesia personnel.[40]

The clinical picture of brainstem anesthesia is protean in manifestation[33,41] producing signs which vary[33] from mild confusion,[31] through marked shivering[42] or convulsions[31], bilateral brainstem nerve palsies (including motor nerve blocking to the contralateral orbit with amaurosis)[43-46] or hemi-, para-, or quadriplegia,[31] with or without loss of consciousness, to apnea with marked cardiovascular instability.[15,23,24] Two patients given posterior peribulbar blocks experienced brainstem anesthesia including apnea.[47]

Central spread should be suspected if there is onset of any of the following:
1. Mental confusion or loss of contact with patient
2. Signs of extraocular paresis or amaurosis of the contralateral eye
3. Shivering bordering on convulsant behavior
4. Nausea/vomiting
5. Dysphagia
6. Sudden swings in the cardiovascular vital signs
7. Dyspnea or respiratory depression.

These signs may be present in various arrangements, e.g. the apneic patient may be conscious, or contralateral eye signs may be the only abnormality detected in an otherwise uneventful block. The onset of brainstem anesthesia should be suspected if there is any indication of loss of patient contact. Ahn and Stanley emphasize the frequent finding of signs of central spread on examination of the contralateral orbit as one of the earliest evidences of the syndrome.[31] If the patient is still conscious, amaurosis may be reported. Usually the contralateral pupil is dilated and areflexic. Oculomotor palsies or frank paralyses may be present in any combination.

On confirmation that spread has affected the opposite eye, the physician should immediately be prepared for progression to any degree of development of the syndrome and be ready to provide support including cardiopulmonary resuscitation; where this is instituted a favorable outcome is the rule. Should recognition be delayed then serious sequelae including death can result. Routine pulse oximetric monitoring of oxygen saturation is valuable and desirable in the block and operating rooms.[32] It should be mandatory whenever a large volume of anesthetic or a very deep needle insertion is used.

Treatment of central spread includes ventilatory support with oxygen, intravenous fluid therapy, and positioning and pharmacologic circulatory support with vagolytics, vasopressors, vasodilators or adrenergic blocking agents as dictated by close vital sign monitoring.

Cardiac arrest has been reported in three papers;[26,36,48] one case required cardiopulmonary resuscitation lasting 45 minutes. In animal experiments direct application of local anesthetics, particularly bupivacaine, to specific areas of the brain had a profound effect on myocardial function.[49,50] Marked increases in arterial blood pressure and heart rate have been reported with brainstem anesthesia[22-24,26,29,36,51,52] which in two cases progressed to pulmonary edema.[23,51]

Hamilton, using a 38 mm (1 1/2") 27 gauge disposable needle observed 20 episodes of central spread in more than 16,000 administrations.[41] From subsequent experience with 5,000 cataract surgeries under local anesthesia using a 32 mm (1 1/4") needle and precision placement (as described in Chapter Three) brainstem anesthesia has not been repeated. Presumably the 38-mm needle had the additional length to pierce the optic nerve sheath. No patient experienced loss of vision, therefore, the needle probably did not penetrate the dura in the apex of the orbit.

The dural sheath covering the intraorbital portion of the optic nerve is not impervious to anesthetic as evidenced by the high incidence of amaurosis following retrobulbar block.

The optic nerve has not been directly examined following cases of brainstem anesthesia and there is no reported incidence of obvious optic nerve trauma, such as optic neuropathy or nerve sheath hemorrhage following the occurrence of brainstem anesthesia. In fact, in cases of needle trauma to the optic nerve in which subsheath bleeding was evident, a different clinical picture was seen and in this circumstance central spread was not reported.[34,53,54]

Brainstem anesthesia has been reported when the injectate did not contain hyaluronidase, therefore, this enzyme does not seem to cause the complication.[31,36]

Much is known about prevention of this syndrome. Unsold et al in 1981 exposed the danger of the elevated, adducted globe during inferotemporal needle placement.[55] This position places the optic nerve in closer proximity to the advancing needle. With the globe in primary gaze, which is advocated, the nerve is less vulnerable. Avoidance of deep penetration of the orbit in any technique is advisable both to prevent this and other serious block complications. Katsev et al advised that maximum penetration from the orbit rim should be 31 mm.[56] In the presence of resistance, injection should be withheld and the needle tip relocated.[36] Modern techniques avoid deep orbital placement and instead advocate accurate injection at limited orbital depth and using increased volume of injectate to achieve critical blocking concentration at the apex.[41]

Brainstem anesthesia has been reported with the curved needle technique when the needle point should have been no further than 5 mm behind the hind surface of the eye.

Ocular Penetration and Perforation

The term penetration is used to indicate needle entry though the scleral coat of the globe, while the term perforation indicates both entry into and exit from the globe during attempted safe needle placement.[57] To avoid serious incidents of this type, the importance of block technique, needle length and type, and modifying technique for myopic patients is stressed.

Such complications are more likely in patients with elongated myopic eyes. Patients presenting for retinal detachment and radial keratotomy surgery tend to have longer globes than patients requiring cataract surgery.[58] Particularly at risk are myopic patients with staphyloma.[59]

Reports of ocular penetration and perforation in the literature range from none in a series of 2,000 peribulbar anesthesias[60] through one in a series of 12,000 comprising both peri- and retrobulbar,[32] and one in a series of 1,000,[61] to three in a series of 4,000 retrobulbar blocks.[58] There are many case reports of the complication including its occurrence with the peribulbar method.[47,62-66] Topical and limbal anesthesia methods have been introduced in an attempt to overcome serious complications related to regional anesthesia for ophthalmology, including scleral perforation.[67] Nevertheless, anterior eyewall perforation has been reported with the method[68] and incomplete anesthesia has been seen.[69] Because these techniques have no way to control the position of the globe if intraoperative complications occur, most cataract surgeons remain skeptical of the methods.[70]

There are four tenets to follow for globe safety: (1) knowledge of axial length and size of the globe; (2) eyes open so that movement of the globe can be recognized; (3) protection of the globe superiorly and inferiorly by overhanging bone; (4) knowledge that pushing on the globe anterior to the equator may rotate the posterior pole into the path of a needle.

In cataract surgery a precise axial length measurement is usually available to determine intraocular lens power calculations. There is higher risk of injury in longer than average eyes which usually have a greater equatorial diameter. When the axial length is not precisely known, knowledge of the dioptric power of their spectacles or contact lenses provides valuable clues to globe dimensions in myopic patients.

Fine disposable needles, which are less painful, are safe, however, excellent anatomic knowledge of the orbit is essential. Grizzard et al reporting on iatrogenic ocular perforation, found that serious injury is much greater with the use of larger dull needles than with fine disposable ones.[63]

Penetration may be suspected in the presence of hypotony, poor red reflex, vitreous hemorrhage and "poking through sensation".[71] The patient may report pain at the time of the perforation,[72] particularly if anesthetic is injected intraocularly. Indirect fundoscopy confirms the diagnosis if the media are sufficiently clear.

Retinal detachment is a common sequela of this complication, calling for appropriate reattachment surgery to prevent visual loss. For appropriate management of scleral perforation and its possible sequelae, the reader is referred to the papers by Feibel,[37] Ramsay and Knoblock[58] and Rinkoff, Doft and Lobes.[57]

Retrobulbar Hemorrhage, Retinal Vascular Occlusion, Optic Nerve Trauma and Late Optic Atrophy

Retrobulbar hemorrhages vary in severity. Some are venous and spread slowly. Signs of severe arterial hemorrhage include a rapid and taut orbital swelling, marked proptosis with immobility of the globe and massive blood staining of the lids and conjunctiva.[37] Serious impairment of the vascular supply to the globe may result.[73,74] Vigilance and keen observation of the signs immediately following needle withdrawal may minimize bleeding. Rapid application of digital pressure over a gauze pad applied to the closed lids may confine it.

The incidence of serious retrobulbar bleeding is reported as 1% to 3%.[75] Undoubtedly with traditional techniques, using 22 and 23 gauge dull needles directed deeply toward the apex, vessels may not have been easily penetrated, but when this occurred serious bleeding could rapidly ensue. A strong argument in favor of fine disposable needles over those of larger gauge[32,76] is that if a vessel is perforated, then a smaller and less precipitous amount of bleeding will occur through a small rent. Additionally, small needle techniques require little or no sedation. Patients experience decreased pain during the administration.

To reduce bleeding, needle insertion must be avoided in the more vascular areas of the orbit. The apex contains the largest vessels entering and exiting the orbit. When serious bleeding occurs here the problem of general orbital pressure increases making surgery difficult,[10] as does the potential obstruction of the globe's blood supply, with resultant compromise of the retinal circulation.

Investigation of retrobulbar hemorrhage includes intraocular pressure measurement, and ophthalmoscopy to check the retinal circulation, if the media are sufficiently clear. Management may include osmotic diuresis,[10] anterior paracentesis to lower intraocular pressure although this is somewhat controversial,[37] and lateral canthotomy for blood drainage or more extensive surgical decompression of the orbit.[37,77]

Klein et al and Cowley et al reported retinal vascular occlusion in the absence of retrobulbar hemorrhage following retrobulbar injection of local anesthetics in patients with severe hematologic or vascular disorders. They postulated trauma to the central retinal artery, or pharmacologic or compressive effects of the injected solution as the cause.[53,78]

Frank optic nerve injury after retrobulbar injection of anesthetic agents may occur along with serious compromise of the globe's blood supply. Computerized scanning or ultrasonography may reveal a dilated optic nerve sheath suggesting intrasheath hemorrhage.[54,76,79] The retinal fundus appearance following an intrasheath injection may resemble Purtscher's retinopathy, a condition thought to be related to rapid elevation of venous pressure.[76,80] Surgical decompression of the nerve sheath may be indicated.

In some cases the increased orbital pressure of retrobulbar hemorrhage may tamponade the small nutrient vessels in the optic nerve, explaining those cases of profound visual loss in which retinal vascular occlusion was not seen and late optic atrophy developed.[37] Other factors in cases of this latter type may be postoperative glaucoma[81] and preexisting small vessel disease such as diabetes. However not all cases of late optic atrophy are easily explainable.[82] Jarrett and Brockhurst reported eleven cases of unexplained optic atrophy following scleral buckling under general anesthesia.[83]

Minor Bleeding Phenomena

The anterior orbit has smaller vessels than exist posteriorly. Three anterior orbital locations are relatively avascular: the inferotemporal quadrant, superotemporally in the sagittal plane of the lateral limbus, and the compartment that is on the nasal side of the medial rectus muscle. Small needles (27 and 30 gauge) placed in these three locations by

Hamilton reduces minor bleeding (including retro-, and peribulbar hemorrhages, subconjunctival bleeding and lid ecchymoses) from a published incidence of 2.75%[32] to 1.0%. The superonasal area should be avoided.

Lid ecchymosis is one of the most disconcerting cosmetic sequelae of retrobulbar or peribulbar anesthesia.[84] This can be largely eliminated using the described relatively avascular areas for needle placement.

Intravascular Injection

Aldrete et al[4] have established that retrograde arterial flow of anesthetic can produce convulsions and cardiovascular collapse in animals and hypothesize that to be the cause of a similar reaction in the human. Slow injection of anesthetic solution eliminates this complication.

Rapid intravenous injection of local anesthetic can cause dangerously high levels in the brain or myocardium from even the small dosage used in ophthalmic anesthesia. Therefore, slow injection of anesthetic in the orbit is mandatory.

Steroid and Antibiotic Injections

Orbital injections of depot steroid medications and antibiotics are frequently employed at the time of ophthalmic surgery for their anti-inflammatory and anti-injective properties. Inadvertent injection of either type into the vitreous has serious implications.[85] Caution is indicated in delivering steroids and antibiotics in a planned extraocular location, to avoid intravascular placement of the needle tip. Aspiration prior to injection is advised. There are many reports of retinal ciliary arterial embolism of these medications, some with irreversible vision deterioration.[75,86-89] On the other hand, the intraocular injection of anesthetics appears to be better tolerated.[37,90,91]

Non-Ptosis Extraocular Muscle Malfunction

Prolonged extraocular muscle malfunction may follow regional anesthesia of the orbit.[19,32] Diplopia and ptosis are common 24 to 48 hours postoperatively when long acting local anesthesia drugs have been used in large volume, indicating the protein binding properties of these agents.[84] Persistence, however, or failure to recover indicates toxic change within the muscle or damage to the nerve supply. When muscle recovery is delayed more than six weeks, 25% of patients suffer permanent damage.[92] It is a complication of the greatest magnitude for a patient to have a perfect optical result and end up with diplopia.

Animal and human investigations of myotoxicity of local anesthetics have been published.[68,93-95] Admixtures with epinephrine may accentuate the problem.[94,95] Several papers stress the importance of avoiding injection into any of the delicate orbital muscles.[3,94-96] Higher concentrations of agents are more likely to result in myotoxicity.[68]

However, it is worth repeating that the more common cause of prolonged muscle malfunction, whatever concentration of local anesthetic is used, is intramuscular injection; this usually clears in two to three weeks, if the nerve has not been damaged.[57] It is imperative to have a good three dimensional knowledge of the anatomy of the orbit and its contents to avoid muscles and nerves.

Postoperative Ptosis

Ptosis is common and as inevitable as the development of cataracts.[97] If defined as a drop of the eyelid margin lower than 2 mm from the superior limbus, then the incidence of ptosis as pre-existing before cataract surgery is reported in 55.5%[98] and 67%[97] of patients. Most postcataract ptosis occurs in patients in whom the levator aponeurosis is already unhealthy (Darrel E. Wolfley, MD, Washington, DC, personal communication). Degenerative conditions of the aponeurosis include disinsertion in the tarsal plate, dehiscence and rarefaction.[97,99,100] Many of these lids would have become ptotic even without cataract surgery. The surgery only serves to accelerate a pre-existing condition (Darrel E. Wolfley, MD, Washington, DC, personal communication).

Extension of pre-existing ptosis, or first time appearance, can occur after cataract, anterior or posterior segment, or orbital and oculoplastic surgery.[97] The published incidence varies from 0% through 20%.[97-99] A lower incidence of postoperative ptosis is seen in surgeries done under general rather than local anesthesia.[99,101] Surgical repair of postoperative ptosis may be necessary if vision is affected, but should be delayed six months until a stable state has been reached.[98,99]

Kaplan et al list many factors that may be involved in the production of postoperative ptosis.[98] These include edema of the eyelid caused by the local anesthesia or following surgery; effects from pressure applied to the globe and upper lid; pressure exerted by the lid speculum; traction on the superior rectus muscle complex from the bridle suture; and prolonged postoperative patching.

They studied 456 patients and concluded that trauma to the superior rectus muscle complex by the bridle suture was the most critical factor in postoperative ptosis. These workers also found that at six months postoperatively the degree of ptosis receded from its immediate postoperative state in 12% of patients. Deady et al, however, did not find any evidence of progressive ptosis.[99] Rainin and Carlson theorize that toxic damage to muscle fibres from direct intramuscular injection of local anesthetics may account for many cases of transient and permanent ptosis.[95]

The eyelid crease is higher in the presence of ptosis. It is prudent to routinely chart eyelid margin height on the cornea and eyelid crease positions including close-up photography bilaterally before surgery. Patients should be informed of the possibility of eyelids drooping temporarily or permanently after surgery. Written consent acknowledging this complication should be obtained.

Orbital Decompression Devices

Orbital decompression devices are essential to prepare the eye for surgery after the use of modern high volume regional anesthesia. Atkinson stressed the importance of the "soft eye" in avoiding complications, particularly vitreous loss.[7,102] In young individuals with low scleral rigidity and greater orbital pressure it is prudent to add pharmacologically induced osmotic diuresis, for example, intravenous mannitol, to achieve optimal operating conditions.

Phacoemulsification techniques, which require a shorter scleral incision, can be used with greater safety in the presence of vitreous pressure than intracapsular or regular extracapsular methods. Decompression promotes akinesia of the periorbital muscles by displacing the anesthetic mixture from within the orbit into the region of the orbicularis muscle thus avoiding a separate and painful seventh nerve block.[77] Pressure on the eyelid may be a factor in the production of postoperative ptosis.[98]

Many types of orbital decompression devices are available.[103-106] Otto and Spekreijse in an animal model studied the effect on intra-orbital pressure of volume discrepancies in the orbit.[100] With decompression devices the major drop in pressure occurs in the first 10 minutes and at a slower rate thereafter, 30 to 45 minutes from the initial block seems ideal. Although decompression devices have been used in large numbers of patients with apparent safety, research into their acute and long-term effects on the retinal circulation would be reassuring. Reduced compression time or force may be appropriate for patients with suspected retinal or optic nerve vascular problems.

Corneal Injury

Care must be taken to protect the cornea in the perioperative period. An occlusive dressing should be used after surgery to seal the eyelids until motor function has returned. This time depends mainly on the duration of action of the chosen anesthetic. Until a safe protocol of dressing management is established occasional corneal exposure may be seen. Prolonged patching may contribute to the production of ptosis.[98]

Possibly the moist atmosphere beneath a gauze pad provides an ideal culture medium for organism growth.[107] "Some experienced surgeons feel it is unnecessary to patch the eye postoperatively"[84] but this decision, from the viewpoint of risk of superficial corneal damage, depends on the degree of lid akinesia in that surgeon's technique. Regional anesthesia can suppress lacrimal gland function making the cornea more susceptible to damage.[68,93]

Oculocardiac Reflex

Meyers states that oculo-cardiac reflex is the most common complication of retrobulbar block.[4] Hamilton has not seen this in over 25,000 administrations either during the blocks, after application of the orbital decompression device or intraoperatively. Hustead has not seen it in 20,000 cases; however in a published series of 12,000 cases a 0.5 and 0.85 percent incidence of vasovagal activity (twice as common in men than in women) was seen. It occurred in patients with a history of fainting.[32] Nicoll et al report similar results based on a series of 6,000 patients.[36] It may be that dull, larger gauge needles and their rapid rate of injection caused this complication in the reported series. Ellis reports that retrobulbar hemorrhage may initiate an oculo-cardiac reflex.[87]

Intraoperative and Postoperative Pain

Comparing traditional low volume with high volume techniques, Hamilton reported a 20 times reduction in the incidence of pain during surgery, from 2.1% to 0.1%.[32] With the recently described limbal anesthesia method,[67] which employs a small volume of anesthetic and does not aim for globe akinesia, it is not surprising that patients may experience pain.[69]

It is common to administer antibiotic by subconjunctival injection at the end of surgery. This often results in considerable pain and may result in site irritation postoperatively. Friedberg et al described a simple painless technique in which the antibiotic is given at the commencement of surgery.[108] As a painless alternative, antibiotics may be injected intraocularly at the time of surgery, using appropriately diluted preparations (H.V. Gimbel, personal communication).

Modern surgical techniques provide minimal tissue disruption and minimal postoperative discomfort after the local anesthetic has worn off; Livingston et al have advocated that short acting agents are sufficient for routine practice.[109] However, the patients are noticeably more comfortable with a small concentration of bupivacaine in the anesthetic mixture. High concentrations of bupivacaine or etidocaine for routine cataract surgery are probably best avoided because of the incidence of diplopia at 24 hours, risk of corneal abrasion and potentiation of ptosis with prolonged patching. For more prolonged surgeries, the use of long acting agents is desirable.

Suprachoroidal Hemorrhage

Choroidal bleeding may occur under general or regional anesthesia and may be spontaneous. It may be precipitated by "bucking," coughing or sneezing, or restlessness from a full urinary bladder. Preoperative arterial hypertension should be reasonably controlled before intraocular surgery. Blood pressure higher than 180/110[110] indicates that surgery should be postponed until the pressure is controlled. Sublingual nifedipine 10 mg, which may be repeated once, is effective in controlling the acute situation.

Phacoemulsification's smaller incisions allow this form of bleeding to be more easily controlled.[111] Intravenous lidocaine is the drug of choice in managing persistent cough in bronchitic patients for whom regional anesthesia is the chosen method.[112,113] Deep breathing exercises, chest physiotherapy, and teaching such patients to control coughing may be even more beneficial. An announced short cough from the lung full position does not raise intraocular pressure.

Use of Anticoagulants

It has been common practice in all types of surgery to reduce or discontinue anticoagulant therapy prior to an operation. The safety of this action for the cataract surgery patient, has been questioned.[114,115] Robinson and Nylander further support the stance that the risk of stopping anticoagulants for this type of surgery is greater than any risk imposed by their continuance.[116] It seems prudent to pay particular attention to the use of fine needle injections in avascular areas when these cases are done with regional anesthesia.

Post Cataract-Extraction Atonic Pupil Syndrome

Postoperative atonic pupil syndrome is a rare complication of cataract surgery. Friedberg reported direct damage from a retrobulbar needle to the ciliary ganglion or adjacent parasympathetic nerve fibres as the probable mechanism.[117] Lam et al reported on seven cases of this syndrome, in which they postulated the iris sphincter as the lesion site, and described a pilocarpine test that eliminated needle trauma to the ciliary ganglion (or other neurogenic etiology) in all seven.[118]

Topical Concerns

While topical anesthesia bears none of the attendant risks associated with regional block anesthesia, there are situations in which the surgeon may need to convert to injected anesthesia. Indications for conversion include the small number of patients who are photophobic. These individuals will be unable to tolerate the microscope light and should be immediately converted to regional anesthesia.

Those patients who cannot comply with instructions to look down or who complain of discomfort should be converted to regional anesthesia, although, dependent on surgical skill, some of these cases may be completed under topical anesthesia. Patients who complain of discomfort from iris chafing should be converted to regional anesthesia.

If a burning sensation exists at the beginning of or during the procedure, additional anesthetic drops may be required. If the patient feels any stinging sensation from the drops instilled in the operating room prior to surgery after the initial drops in the preoperative area, then the effectiveness of the topical drop should be determined.

To avoid potential complications with topical anesthesia, patients should never be oversedated either pre- or intraoperatively because they will be unable to fully cooperate with the surgeon's instructions. Also, if a bridle suture is necessary to control eye movement, additional anesthesia will be needed in the form of a subconjunctival injection. Also pain may be experienced due to over-expansion of the anterior chamber, therefore normal hydraulic control is important.

Summary

Complications of regional anesthesia for ophthalmology can be minimized by performing blocks with fine gauge disposable needles, precisely positioned in relatively avascular areas at limited depth, avoiding extraocular muscles. By using adequate volumes of anesthetic agents injected through needles thus placed, safe and effective anesthesia and ocular akinesia are achieved.

Primary gaze directioning during all needle placements and alignment of needles tangentially to the globe is critical. Percutaneous seventh nerve blocking can be avoided. Training of practitioners in the art and science of ophthalmic regional anesthesia should be done by personnel with extensive experience and knowledge. With clearly defined guidelines, regional anesthesia for intraocular surgery can be made virtually foolproof. However, one must always remember that "it is impossible to make anything foolproof because fools are so ingenious."[119]

What has become clear in the evolution of ophthalmic anesthesia is that open communication among clinicians plays a critically important role in stimulating progress. It is this generous sharing of ideas, research, and actual clinical data, and the willingness to learn from the positive and negative experiences that will provide the impetus for ophthalmologists, anesthetists and researchers to develop better ways to serve the most important person in this whole equation—the patient.

References

1. Rubin AP. Anaesthesia for cataract surgery - time for change? Editorial. Anaesthesia 1990;45:717-8.
2. Zeitlin GL, Hobin K, Platt J, Woitkoski N. Accumulation of carbon dioxide during eye surgery. J Clin Anesth 1989;1:262-7.
3. O'Brien CS. Local anesthesia. Archiv Ophthalmol 1934;12:240-53.

6. Havener WH. Hand-holding anesthesia. Ophthalmic Surg 1990;21:375-6.
7. Atkinson WS. Akinesia of the orbicularis. Am J Ophthalmol 1953;36:1255-8.
8. Feibel RM. Robert E. Wright and the development of facial nerve akinesia. Surv Ophthalmol 1989;33:523-8.
9. Nadbath RP, Rehman I. Facial nerve block. Amer J Ophthalmol 1963;55:143-6.
10. Olander KW, in Masket S (ed). Consultation section. J Cataract Refract Surg 1990;16:766-74.
11. van Lint. Paralysie palpebral temporaire provoquee dans l'operation de la cataracte. Ann d'Ocul 1914;151:420-4.
12. Wright RE. Blocking of the main trunk of the facial nerve in cataract operations. Arch Ophthalmol 1926;55:555-9.
13. Koenig SB, Snyder RW, Kay J. Respiratory distress after a Nadbath block. Ophthalmology 1988;95:1285-7.
14. Lindquist TD, Kopietz LA, Spigelman AV, et al. Complications of Nadbath facial nerve block and review of the literature. Ophthalmic Surg 1988;19:271-3.
15. Ruusuvaara P, Setala K, Tarkkanen A. Respiratory arrest after retrobulbar block. Acta Ophthalmol 1988;66:223-5.
16. Spaeth GL. Total facial nerve palsy following modified O'Brien facial nerve block. Ophthalmic Surg 1987;18:518-9.
17. Hamilton RC. Brainstem anesthesia as a complication of regional anesthesia for ophthalmology. Can J Ophthalmol 1992 (in press).
18. Kaufer G, Augustin G. Orbitography: Report of a complication with use of water-soluble contrast material. Am J Ophthalmol 1966;61:795-8.
19. Rao VA, Kawatra VK. Ocular myotoxic effects of local anesthetics. Can J Ophthalmol 1988;23:171-3.
20. Drysdale DB. Experimental subdural retrobulbar injection of anesthetic. Ann Ophthalmol 1984;16:716-8.
21. Wang BC, Bogart B, Hillman DE, Turndorf H. Subarachnoid injection - a potential complication of retrobulbar block. Anesthesiology 1989;71:845-7.
22. Beltranean HP, Vega MJ, Kirk N, Blankenship G. Inadvertent intravascular bupivacaine injection following retrobulbar block. Reg Anesth 1981;6:149-151.
23. Chang J-L, Gonzalez-Abola E, Larson CE, Lobes L. Brain stem anesthesia following retrobulbar block. Anesthesiology 1984;61:789-90.
24. Hamilton RC. Brain stem anesthesia following retrobulbar blockade. Anesthesiology 1985;63:688-90.
25. Mercereau DA. Brain-stem anesthesia complicating retrobulbar block. Can J Ophthalmol 1989;24:159-61.
26. Rosenblatt RM, May DR, Barsoumian K. Cardiopulmonary arrest after retrobulbar block. Amer J Ophthalmol 1980;90:425-7.
27. Smith JL. Retrobulbar Marcaine can cause respiratory arrest. J Clin Neuro-Ophthalmol 1981;1:171-2.
28. Aldrete JA, Romo-Salas F, Arora S, Wilson R, Rutherford R. Reverse arterial blood flow as a pathway for central nervous system toxic responses following injection of local anesthetics. Anesth Analg 1978; 57:428-33.
29. Javitt JC, Addiego R, Friedberg HL, Libonati MM, Leahy JJ. Brain stem anesthesia after retrobulbar block. Ophthalmology 1987;94:718-24.
30. Kobet KA. Cerebral spinal fluid recovery of lidocaine and bupivacaine following respiratory arrest subsequent to retrobulbar block. Ophthalmic Surg 1987;18:11-3.
31. Ahn JC, Stanley JA. Subarachnoid injection as a complication of retrobulbar anesthesia. Amer J Ophthalmol 1987;103:225-30.
32. Hamilton RC, Gimbel HV, Strunin L. Regional anesthesia for 12,000 cataract extraction and intraocular lens implantation procedures. Can J Anaesth 1988;35:615-23.
33. Nicoll JMV, Acharya PA, Edge KR, et al. Shivering following retrobulbar block. Can J Anaesth 1988;35:671.
34. Stanley JA. Subarachnoid injection of retrobulbar anesthetic as a complication of retrobulbar block. Saudi Bull Ophthalmol 1987;2:13-7.
35. Wittpenn JR, Rapoza P, Sternberg P, Kuwashima L, Saklad J, Patz A. Respiratory arrest following retrobulbar anesthesia. Ophthalmology 1986;93:867-70.
36. Nicoll JMV, Acharya PA, Ahlen K, et al. Central nervous system complications after 6000 retrobulbar blocks. Anesth Analg 1987;66:1298-1302.
37. Feibel RM. Current concepts in retrobulbar anesthesia. Surv Ophthalmol 1985;30:102-10.
38. Kaplan SL. Peribulbar anesthesia. Ophthalmic Surg 1988;19:374.
39. Morgan GE. Retrobulbar apnea syndrome: A case for the routine presence of an anesthesiologist. Reg Anesth 1990;15:107.
40. Leaming DV. Practice styles and preferences of ASCRS members - 1989 survey. J Cataract Refract Surg 1990;16:624-32.

41. Hamilton RC, Gimbel HV, Javitt JC. The prevention of complications of regional anesthesia for ophthalmology. In: Zahl K, Meltzer MA, eds. Ophthalmol Clin N Amer: Regional anesthesia for intraocular surgery. WB Saunders, 1990:pp111-25.

42. Lee DS, Kwon NJ. Shivering following retrobulbar block. Can J Anaesth 1988;35:294-6.

43. Antoszyk AN, Buckley EG. Contralateral decreased visual acuity and extraocular muscle palsies following retrobulbar anesthesia. Ophthalmology 1986;93:462-5.

44. Follette JW, LoCascio JA. Bilateral amaurosis following unilateral retrobulbar block. Anesthesiology 1985;63:237-8.

45. Friedberg HL, Kline OR. Contralateral amaurosis after retrobulbar injection. Amer J Ophthalmol 1986;101:668-90.

46. Rogers R, Orellana J. Cranial nerve palsy following retrobulbar anesthesia. Brit J Ophthalmol 1988;72:78.

47. Davis DB, Mandel MR. Peribulbar: reducing complications. Ocular Surg News 1989;7:21.

48. Cardan E, Pop R, Negrutiu S. Prolonged haemodynamic disturbance following attempted retrobulbar block. Anaesthesia 1987;42:668-9.

49. Heavner JE. Cardiac dysrhythmias induced by infusion of local anesthetics into the lateral cerebral ventricle of cats. Anesth Analg 1986;65:133-8.

50. Thomas RD, Behbehani MM, Coyle DE, Denson DD. Cardiovascular toxicity of local anesthetics: an alternative hypothesis. Anesth Analg 1986;65:444-50.

51. Elk JR, Wood J, Holladay JT. Pulmonary edema following retrobulbar block. J Cataract Refract Surg 1988;14:216-7.

52. Nique TA, Bennet CA. Inadvertent brain stem anesthesia following extra-oral trigeminal V2-V3 blocks. Oral Surg 1981;51:468-70.

53. Klein ML, Jampol LM, Condon PI, et al. Central retinal artery occlusion without retrobulbar hemorrhage after retrobulbar anesthesia. Am J Ophthalmol 1982;93:573-7.

54. Sullivan KL, Brown GC, Forman AR, et al. Retrobulbar anesthesia and retinal vascular obstruction. Ophthalmology 1983;90:373-7.

55. Unsold R, Stanley JA, DeGroot J. The CT-topography of retrobulbar anesthesia. Graefes Arch Clin Exp Ophthalmol 1981;217:125-36.

56. Katsev DA, Drews RC, Rose BT. An anatomic study of retrobulbar needle path length. Ophthalmology 1989;96:1221-4.

57. Rinkoff JS, Doft BH, Lobes LA. Management of ocular penetration from injection of local anesthesia preceding cataract surgery. Arch Ophthalmol 1991;109:1421-5.

58. Ramsay RC, Knobloch WH. Ocular perforation following retrobulbar anesthesia for retinal detachment surgery. Am J Ophthalmol 1978;86:61-4.

59. Rosen DA. Anesthesia in ophthalmology. Can Anaesth Soc J 1962;9:545-9.

60. Davis DB, Mandel MR. Posterior peribulbar anesthesia: An alternative to retrobulbar anesthesia. J Cataract Refract Surg 1986;12:182-4.

61. Cibis PA. Discussion in Schepens CL, Regan CDJ, (eds): Controversial aspects of the management of retinal detachments. Boston, Little, Brown, 1965, p251.

62. Duker JS, Belmont JB, Benson WE, et al. Inadvertent globe perforation during retrobulbar and peribulbar anesthesia. Ophthalmology 1991;98:519-26.

63. Grizzard WS, Kirk NM, Pavan PR, et al. Perforating ocular injuries caused by anesthesia personnel. Ophthalmology 1991;98:1011-6.

64. Kimble JA, Morris RE, Witherspoon CD, Feist RM. Globe perforation from peribulbar injection. Arch Ophthalmol 1987;105:749.

65. Straus JG. A new retrobulbar needle and injection technique. Ophthalmic Surg 1988;19:134-9.

66. Zaturansky B, Hyams S. Perforation of the globe during the injection of local anesthesia. Ophthalmic Surg 1987;18:585-8.

67. Furuta M, Toriumi T, Kashiwagi K, Satoh S. Limbal anesthesia for cataract surgery. Ophthalmic Surg 1990;21:22-5.

68. Yagiela JA, Benoit PW, Buoncristiani RD, et al. Comparison of myotoxic effects of lidocaine with epinephrine in rats and humans. Anesth Analg 1981;60:471-80.

69. Levin ML, in Masket S (ed). Consultation section. J Cataract Refract Surg 1990;16:766-74.

70. Aquavella JV. Comment (Limbal anesthesia for cataract surgery). Ophthalmic Surg 1990;21:26.

71. Schneider ME, Milstein DE, Oyakawa RT, et al. Ocular perforation from a retrobulbar injection. Amer J Ophthalmol 1988;106:35-40.

72. Seelenfreund MH, Freilich DB. Retinal injuries associated with cataract surgery. Am J Ophthalmol

1980;89:654-8.

73. Goldsmith MO. Occlusion of the central retinal artery following retrobulbar anesthesia. Ophthalmologica 1967;153:191-6.

74. Kraushar MF, Seelenfreund MH, Freilich DB. Central retinal artery closure during orbital hemorrhage from retrobulbar injection. Trans Am Acad Ophthalmol Otolaryngol 1974;78:65-70.

75. Morgan CM, Schatz H, Vine AK, et al. Ocular complications associated with retrobulbar injections. Ophthalmology 1988;95:660-5.

76. Grizzard WS. Ophthalmic anesthesia. In: Reinecke RD, ed. Ophthalmology Annual 1989. Raven Press 1989:pp265-94.

77. McFarland M, in Masket S (ed). Consultation section. J Cataract Refract Surg 1990;16:766-74.

78. Cowley M, Campochiara PA, Newman SA, et al. Retinal vascular occlusion without retrobulbar or optic sheath hemorrhage after retrobulbar injection of lidocaine. Ophthalmic Surg 1988;19:859-61.

79. Hersch M, Baer G, Dieckert JP, et al. Optic nerve enlargement and central retinal-artery occlusion secondary to retrobulbar anesthesia. Ann Ophthalmol 1989;21:195-7.

80. Lemagne J-M, Michiels X, Van Causenbroech S, Snyers B. Purtscher-like retinopathy after retrobulbar anesthesia. Ophthalmology 1990;97:859-61.

81. Hayreh SS. Anterior ischemic optic neuropathy IV. Occurrence after cataract extraction. Arch Ophthalmol 1980;98:1410-6.

82. Carroll FD. Optic nerve complications of cataract extraction. Trans Am Acad Ophthalmol Otolaryngol 1973;77:623-9.

83. Jarrett WH, Brockhurst RJ. Unexplained blindness and optic atrophy following retinal detachment surgery. Arch Ophthalmol 1965;73:782-91.

84. Wallace RB, in Masket S (ed). Consultation section. J Cataract Refract Surg 1990;16:766-74.

85. Schlaegal TF, Wilson FM. Accidental intraocular injection of depot corticosteroids. Trans Am Acad Ophthalmol Otolaryngol 1974;78:847-55.

86. Byers B. Blindness secondary to steroid injections into the nasal turbinates. Arch Ophthalmol 1979; 97:79-80.

87. Ellis PP. Occlusion of the central retinal artery after retrobulbar corticosteroid injection. Am J Ophthalmol 1978;85:352-6.

88. McLean EB. Inadvertent injection of corticosteroid into the choroidal vasculature. Am J Ophthalmol 1975;80:835-7.

89. Shorr N, Seiff SR. Central retinal artery occlusion associated with periocular corticosteroid injection for juvenile hemangioma. Ophthalmic Surg 1986;17:229-31.

90. Berg P, Kroll P, Kuchie HJ. Iatrogenic eye perforations in para- and retrobulbar injections. Klin Monatsbl Augenheilkd 1986;189:170-2.

91. Lincoff H, Zweifach P, Brodie S, et al. Intraocular injection of lidocaine. Ophthalmology 1985;92:1587-91.

92. Tennant JL. Diplopia. Paper read at the 4th Annual Scientific Meeting, Ophthalmic Anesthesia Society, San Antonio, Texas, October 6th, 1990.

93. Carlson BM, Emerick S, Komorowski TE, Rainin EA. Extraocular muscle regeneration in primates. Local anesthesia-induced lesions. Ophthalmology 1992;99:582-9.

94. Foster AH, Carlson BM. Myotoxicity of local anesthetics and regeneration of the damaged muscle fibers. Anesth Analg 1980;59:727-36.

95. Rainin EA, Carlson BM. Postoperative diplopia and ptosis: a clinical hypothesis on the myotoxicity of local anesthetics. Arch Ophthalmol 1985;103:1337-9.

96. Ong-Tone L, Pearce WG. Inferior rectus muscle restriction after retrobulbar anesthesia for cataract extraction. Can J Ophthalmol 1989;24:162-5.

97. Stasior OG. Postoperative ptosis: Etiology, diagnosis, treatment, informed consent. Paper read at the 4th Annual Scientific Meeting, Ophthalmic Anesthesia Society, San Antonio, Texas, October 6th, 1990.

98. Kaplan LJ, Jaffe NS, Clayman HM. Ptosis and cataract surgery. Ophthalmology 1985;92:237-42.

99. Deady JP, Price NJ, Sutton GA. Ptosis following cataract and trabeculotomy surgery. Brit J Ophthalmol 1989;73:283-5.

100. Paris GL, Quickert MH. Disinsertion of the aponeurosis of the levator palpebrae superioris muscle after cataract extraction. Am J Ophthalmol 1976;81:337-40.

101. Alpar JJ. Acquired ptosis following cataract and glaucoma surgery. Glaucoma 1982;4:66-8.

102. Atkinson WS. Observations on anesthesia for ocular surgery. Trans Amer Acad Ophthalmol Otolaryng 1956;60:376-80.

103. Buys NS. Mercury balloon reducer for vitreous and orbital volume control, in Emery J (ed): Current

concepts in cataract surgery. St. Louis, CV Mosby, 1980, p 258.

104. Davidson B, Kratz R, Mazzoco T. An evaluation of the Honan intraocular pressure reducer. Am Intra-ocular Implant Soc J 1979;5:237-8.

105. Drews RC. The Nerf ball for preoperative reduction of intraocular pressure. Ophthalmic Surg 1982;13:761.

106. Gills JP. Constant mild compression of the eye to produce hypotension. Am Intra-ocular Implant Soc J 1979;5:52-3.

107. Laws DE, Watts MT, Kirkby GR, Lawson J. Is padding necessary cataract extraction? Br J Ophthalmol 1989;73:699- 701.

108. Friedberg HL, Kline OR, Galman BD. Painless cataract surgery. J Cataract Refract Surg 1988;14:100.

109. Livingston MW, Mackool RJ, Schneider H. Anesthetic agents used in cataract surgery. J Cataract Refract Surg 1990;16:272.

110. Bloomberg L. Expulsive hemorrhage. Paper read at the 4th Annual Scientific Meeting, Ophthalmic Anesthesia Society, San Antonio, Texas, October 6th, 1990.

111. Welch JC, Spaeth GL, Benson WE. Massive suprachoroidal hemorrhage. Ophthalmology 1988;95:1202-6.

112. Fenton WM. Intravenous lidocaine for control of coughing during standby cataract surgery. Anesthesiology 1986;64:847.

113. Stewart RH, Kimbrough RL, Engstrom PF, et al. Lidocaine: an anti-tussive for ophthalmic surgery. Ophthalmic Surg 1988;19:130-1.

114. Hall DL, Steen WH, Drummond JW, Byrd WA. Anticoagulants and cataract surgery. Ophthalmic Surg 1988;19:221-2.

115. McMahan LB. Anticoagulants and cataract surgery. J Cataract Refract Surg 1988;14:569-71.

116. Robinson GA, Nylander A. Warfarin and cataract extraction. Brit J Ophthalmol 1989;73:702-3.

117. Friedberg HL. Use shorter needle behind globe to avoid persistent mydriasis. Ophthalmol Times 1988;13:16,39.

118. Lam S, Beck RW, Hall D, Creighton JB. Atonic pupil after cataract surgery. Ophthalmology 1989; 96:589-90.

119. Martin TL Jr. Malice in blunderland. New York: McGraw Hill, 1973.

Epilogue

James P. Gills, MD
Robert F. Hustead, MD

PERSPECTIVES

Advances in ophthalmic surgery were rapid after the introduction of general anesthesia in 1846, and mushroomed after the introduction of cocaine for topical anesthesia in 1884. All minor operations, such as foreign bodies or simple cataract, could be done with better surgical results using topical anesthesia. General anesthesia was reserved for the uncooperative patient or for major operations such as complicated cataract, or enucleation. The undesirable morbidity and mortality associated with general anesthesia for these operations were the incentives for the development of regional anesthesia, which produced excellent surgical conditions for simple cataract surgery. Reliable regional anesthesia led to the refinements of surgical technique for cataract surgery of the present decade.

All forms of anesthesia are acceptable which produce zero anesthesia complications and allow the surgeon to produce excellent surgical results. Anesthesia complications can hurt the patient or lead to a less than optimal surgical result. Thus the desirability of an anesthesia technique in ophthalmology can be a measure both of minimal insult to the patient and maximum surgical effectiveness. We question that zero anesthesia morbidity will ever be possible, but it is an end to our continuous striving. As surgical technique for simple cataract have improved during the past decade with smaller incisions, hydraulically sealing wounds, and means to maintain a stable intraocular pressure, there has been increasing concern to reduce the need for regional anesthesia and the morbidity associated with needle injections.

We look forward to the next decade in which controlled studies will establish that optimal surgical correction of ocular disease can occur with no anesthesia morbidity. Should regional anesthesia attempt to maintain its premier position, it must give proper attention to the anatomy of the globe and orbit and to the million little details that permit its optimum safe use.

GUIDE TO FIGURE ABBREVIATIONS

Abbreviations and Acroynms

a—arachnoid
ac—anterior chamber
aea—anterior ethmoid artery
aen—anterior ethmoid nerve
aev—anterior ethmoid vein
an—abducens nerve
atc—adipose tissue compartment
av—angular vein
az—annulus of Zinn
c—cornea
ca—ciliary artery
cg-n—ciliary ganglion
cj—conjunctiva
cjb—bulbar conjunctiva
cjf—conjunctival fornix
cjs—conjunctival sac
cn—ciliary nerve
cns—canthus, nasal
cpal—capsulopalpebral ligament (anterior lamella)
cppl—capsulopalpebral ligament (posterior lamella)
cra—central retinal artery
crv—central retinal vein
cta—cillary artery trunk
ctp—canthus, temporal
d—dura mater
dna—dorsal nasal artery
eb—ethmoid bone
es—ethmoidal sinuses
elic—eyelid, lower, skin crease
ell—eyelid, lower
elu—eyelid, upper
eluc—eyelid, upper, skin crease
fb—frontal bone
fn—frontal nerve

fv—facial vein
fpm—frontal process of the maxilla
g—globe
ibsov—inferior branch of superior ophthalmic vein
ica—internal carotid artery
ima—inferior muscular artery
ioa—infraorbital artery
ioc—infraorbital canal
iof—infraorbital fissure
iom—inferior oblique muscle
ion—infraorbital nerve
ior—inferior orbital rim
iov—inferior ophthalmic vein
irm—inferior rectus muscle
ita—infratrochlear artery
itn—infratrochlear nerve
l—lens
la—lacrimal artery
laal—levator (anterior lamella)
lac—lacrimal crest, anterior
lalf—levator aponeurosis, lateral
lamf—levator aponeurosis, medial
lapl—levator (posterior lamella)
lb—lacrimal bone
lc—lacrimal canal
lci—lacrimal canaliculus, inferior
lcl—lateral check ligament
lcs—lacrimal canaliculus, superior
lct—lateral canthal tendon
lcv—lateral collateral vein
lg—lacrimal gland
lgop—lacrimal gland orbital part
lgpp—lacrimal gland palpebral part
lii—limbus, inferior
lins—limbus, nasal

lis—limbus, superior
litp—limbus, temporal
ll—lacrimal lake
ln—lacrimal nerve
lnabs—lacrimal nerve absent
lol—Lockwood's ligament
lpc—lacrimal crest, posterior
lpca—long posterior ciliary artery
lpl—lateral palpebral ligament
lrm—lateral rectus muscle
ls—lacrimal sack
lsa—lacrimal sack artery
lsn—lacrimal sack nerve
lsv—lacrimal sack vein
lv—lacrimal vein
ma—maxillary artery
mb—maxillary bone
mbfa—meningeal branch of frontal artery
mcl—medial check ligament
mct—medial canthal tendon
mcv—medial collateral vein
mm—Muller's muscle
mn—maxillary nerve
mov—medial ophthalmic vein
mpa—medial palpebral arteries
mpl—medial palpebral ligament
mpv—medial palpebral veins
mrm—medial rectus muscle
mua—muscular artery
muv—muscular vein
nb—nasal bone
ncn—nasociliary nerve
nlc—nasolacrimal canal
nld—nasolacrimal duct
oa—ophthalmic artery
oc—optic canal
ocsp—optic canal, superior pillar
olfv—orbito-lacrimo-facial vein
omc—oculomotor compartment
omin—oculomotor nerve, inferior branch
omn—oculomotor nerve
omsn—oculomotor nerve, superior branch
omv—"veine ophtalmique moyenne"
on—optic nerve
oom—orbicularis oculi muscle
opeb—orbital plate of ethmoid bone
oppb—orbital process of palatine bone
os—orbital septum

ov—ophthalmic vein
p—pia mater
pafp—pre-aponeurptic fat pad
pat—periorbital adipose tissue
pb—palatine bone
pca—posterior ciliary arteries
pcv—posterior collateral vein
pea—posterior ethmoidal artery
pev—posterior ethmoidal vein
pf—periorbital fascia
po—periorbit
pv—pterygoid venous network
s—sclera
sas—subarachnoid space
sb—sphenoid bone
sbsov—superior branch of superior ophthalmic vein
sca—short ciliary artery
slpm—superior levator palpebrae muscle
slpt—superior levator palpebrae tendon
smc—smooth muscle cells
soa—supra-orbital artery
sof—superior orbital fissure
som—superior oblique muscle
son—superior ophthalmic nerve
sor—superior orbital rim
sot—superior oblique tendon
sov—superior ophthalmic vein
srlm—superior rectus/levator muscle complex
srm—superior rectus muscle
sta—supra-trochlear artery
stn—supra-trochlear nerve
stv—supra-trochlear vein
t—trochlea
tc—Tenon's capsule
tm—temporalis muscle
tn—trochlear nerve
tp—tarsal plate
tpi—tarsal plate, inferior
tps—tarsal plate, superior
vv—vortex veins
zb—zygomatic bone
zfa—zygomaticofacial artery
zfc—zygomaticofacial canal
zfn—zygomaticofacial nerve
zpfb—zygomatic process of frontal bone

Major Connective Tissue Septa

1. Connective tissue of the medial rectus muscle attaches to the floor and roof of the orbit.

2. Medial rectus muscle septa communicate and help form the superior ophthalmic vein hammock.

2a. Septum from the temporal surface of the medial rectus muscle to the optic nerve.

3. Septal connections between the medial rectus muscle and the inferior oblique/inferior rectus complex.

4. Connective tissue septa of the inferior oblique muscle which runs parallel to the orbital floor and co-mingles with inferior rectus connective tissue.

5. Septal connections between the inferior oblique muscle and septa of the lateral rectus muscle. The inter-connections form a hammock for the eye known as Lockwood's ligament.

6. Connective tissue septa of the inferior rectus muscle connected with Muller's muscle and the periorbit of the orbital fissure.

7. Connective tissue of the inferior rectus muscle in arch-like septa which surround the muscle and fix it to the infero-lateral orbital wall.

8. Connective tissue of the lateral rectus muscle anchoring it to the lateral orbital wall.

9. The lateral rectus muscle connective tissue attaches it to the inferior oblique connective tissue.

9a. Septa from the nasal aspect of the lateral rectus muscle connecting it to the optic nerve.

10. The lateral rectus muscle connective tissue contribution to the formation of the superior ophthalmic vein hammock.

11. Cranial extensions of the lateral rectus muscle connective tissue blend with the lateral aponeurosis of levator and attach in the area of Whitnall's tubercle.

12. The connective tissue septa of the levator/superior rectus muscle complex connect those muscles to the superior ophthalmic vein forming the medial aspect of the lateral part of the ophthalmic vein hammock. This septum continues laterally to attach the complex to the adjacent periorbit. This septum, as it comes anterior, becomes replaced by a single thick septum, the lateral aponeurosis of the levator muscle. This septum blends with the orbital septum and the tarsal plate and contains smooth muscle fibers in the posterior lamellae.

13. The connective tissue septum of the superior oblique muscle surrounds that muscle and connects it to the periorbit.

Index

Note: Page numbers in *italics* refer to illustrations; numbers followed by (t) indicate tables.